NURSING MADE INSANELY EASY!

Sixth Edition

Sylvia Rayfield, MN, RN, CNS

Loretta Manning, MSN, RN, GNP
President, I CAN Publishing®, Inc.

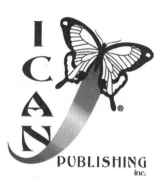

I CAN Publishing®, Inc. ◆ Duluth, GA
www.icanpublishing.com

I CAN Publishing®, Inc., Duluth, GA 30097

2650 Chattahoochee Dr., Suite 100
Duluth, GA 30097
www.icanpublishing.com

Editorial Assistant: Burger Vaughan, Dahlonega, GA;
    Teresa R. Davidson, Greensboro, NC
Cartoon Illustrations: Teresa R. Davidson, Greensboro, NC; Eileen Burke,
    Pass Christian, MS; Paulina Hanson, Words & Pictures; Jeanne Woods,
Design Master, New Orleans, LA; Mitch Rubin, Rubin Art, Albuquerque,
    NM; John Sheppard, Shep Art Studios, Alpharetta, GA
Cover Design: Teresa R. Davidson, Greensboro, NC

ISBN-13: 978-0-9842040-2-1
Library of Congress Catalog Control Number: 2010934281

Nursing procedures and/or practice described in this book should be applied by the nurse or healthcare practitioner under appropriate supervision according to established professional standards of care. These standards should be used with regard to the unique circumstances that apply in each practice situation. Every effort has been taken to validate and confirm the accuracy of information presented and to describe generally accepted practices. However, the authors, editors, and publisher cannot accept any responsibility for errors or omissions or for consequences from application of the information in this book and make no warranty, express or implied, with respect to the contents of this book.

Every effort has been exerted by the authors and publisher to ensure that drug selection and dosage set forth in this text is in accord with current recommendations and practice at the time of publication. However, in view of ongoing research, the constant flow of information relating to governmental regulations, drug therapy, and drug reactions, the reader is urged to check the manufacturer's information on the package insert of each drug for any change in indications and dosage and for added warnings and precautions. This is particularly important when the recommended agent is a new or infrequently used drug.

This book is written to be used as a memory tool (A Visual Approach to Memory) for students, graduates, and faculty. It is not intended for use as a primary resource for procedures, treatments, medications, or to serve as a complete textbook for nursing care. Copies of this book may be obtained directly from I CAN Publishing®, Inc. at www.icanpublishing.com.

In discovering new ways of thinking about nursing concepts and creative ways of helping learners to remember was the reason for writing this book. This is our 6th edition of a book that has sold internationally and helped thousands of learners "get it." We are grateful to our contributors.

Julia Aucoin, DNS, RN-BC, CNE
Chief Knowledge Officer
Practical Success
Durham, NC

Marie Bremner, DSN, RN, CS
Regional Director
NY, PA, and Washington, D.C.
Marietta, GA

Darlene Burke, MS, MA, RN, BC
Faculty
Mira Costa College
Oceanside, CA

Pam Chally, PhD, RN
Dean of the College of Health
University of North Florida
Jacksonville, FL

J. Chris Chandler, BA, BSN, RN
Nursing ADP Coordinator
Atlanta VA Hospital
Decatur, GA

Jo Carol Claborn, MS, RN
Executive Director
Nursing Education Consultants
Dallas, TX

Katherine Crawford, MSN, RN
Case Manager, Quality Management
Shreveport, LA

Martha Eakes, MSN, CNA, RNC
Davidson Community College
Lexington, NC
Administrative Coordinator
Women's Hospital of Greensboro
Greensboro, NC

Shannon D. Foxworth, AD, RN
Florence SC

Melissa J. Geist, APRN, BC, EdD
Assistant Dean
Tennessee Technological University
Cookeville, TN

Alita R. Maddox, APRN,
MSN, PNP-C
In Memory

Karna C. McBrayer, BSN, RN
Educator
Laredo, TX

Jackie McVey, PhD, RN
University of Texas-Tyler
Tyler, TX

Kathy O'Leary Oller, MSN, RN
International Nursing Consultant
Bangladesh
Jacksonville, FL

Tina Rayfield, PA, RN
President
Sylvia Rayfield & Associates, Inc.
Pensacola, FL

Vanice W. Roberts, DSN, RN
Dean of Nursing
Shorter College, Rome, GA

Jessica Roberts, MSN, RN,
Staff Nurse, Emergency Services
North Side Cherokee Hospital
Canton, GA

Bedelia Russell, MSN, RN,
CNOR, CPNP
Assistant Professor
Tennessee Technological University
Cookeville, TN

Martha Sherman, MSN, MA, RN
Retired

Mayola L. Villarruel, RN, MSN, ANP
Director, Patient Care Services
Community Hospital, Munster, IN

JoAnn Zerwekh, EdD, RN, FNP
Executive Director
Nursing Education Consultants
Dallas, TX

OTHER BOOKS PUBLISHED BY I CAN PUBLISHING®, INC.

NCLEX-RN® 101: HOW TO PASS

NCLEX-PN®101: HOW TO PASS

NURSING MADE INSANELY EASY

PHARMACOLOGY MADE INSANELY EASY

PATHWAYS TO TEACHING NURSING: KEEPING IT REAL

WE DO NOT DIE ALONE: "Jesus is Coming to Get Me in a White Pickup Truck"

SEEKING SAFETY: THE JOURNEY OF ADULTS WHO WERE SEXUALLY ABUSED AS CHILDREN

PHARMACOLOGY: NCLEX® REVIEWS

EBOOK

NCLEX® MAKES BIG CHANGES

I CAN Publishing®, Inc.
2650 Chattahoochee Drive, Suite 100
Duluth, GA 30097
1-866-428-5589
www.icanpublishing.com

> *Dedicated with love to nursing students, educators, and practicing nurses in the United States and abroad.*

ACKNOWLEDGMENTS

We wish to express our appreciation to both our families for their never ending support and love, while we developed this book.

- Our families who continue to believe we can do anything.

- Teresa Davidson, our friend, artist, and computer guru.

- The artists that take our words and ideas and interpret them into meaningful and sometimes hilarious images.

- Our contributors (students, teachers, and friends) that see worth in our work and want to be a part of it.

- Our associates in Sylvia Rayfield and Associates, Inc., who make the words and images come to life when they present them in NCLEX® reviews.

- Jennifer Robinson, Administrative Director of I CAN Publishing®, Inc., who is our friend and lifeline in our distribution center.

I
CAN

Did is a word
of achievement,

Won't is a word
of retreat,

Might is a word
of bereavement

Can't is a word
of defeat,

Ought is a word
of duty,

Try is a word
each hour,

Will is a word
of beauty,

Can is a word
of power.

—Author Unknown

"THE IMPORTANT THING IN SCIENCE IS NOT SO MUCH TO OBTAIN NEW FACTS AS TO DISCOVER NEW WAYS OF THINKING ABOUT THEM." ~ Sir William Bragg

CONTENTS

SAFETY AND INFECTION CONTROL

HEALTH PROMOTION

PSYCHOSOCIAL INTEGRITY

SENSORY PERCEPTION

ENDOCRINE

CARDIAC SYSTEM

RESPIRATORY / ACID BASE

FLUID VOLUME / RENAL SYSTEM

MEN & WOMEN'S CARE / CANCER

GASTROINTESTINAL SYSTEM

NEURO / ORTHOPEDIC SYSTEM

PREFACE

A MESSAGE TO OUR LEARNERS

This book was developed to make learning and life easier for student nurses and their teachers in registered and practical nurse programs, graduating nursing students preparing for exit exams, new graduate nurses preparing for NCLEX-RN® and NCLEX-PN® exams, experienced international graduates preparing for the CGFNS® exam and other medical and allied health students that will find it useful.

Our experience with thousands of learners each year has helped us develop images and strategies that accelerate the learning process. The format is insanely easy! On the left page is the "bottom line stuff" about the concept. The image or memory tool is on the right page.

In this 6th edition, we have reorganized the concepts so that the most important (according to National Council of State Boards of Nursing research) comes first in the book. We continue to utilize the acronym SAFETY to provide a way for our learners to organize their clinical and theoretical framework. Many of our images have been updated to reflect changes in current practice.

Many of the most important aspects of nursing are not easily illustrated in visuals. We think these unshown characteristics are a vital part of nursing: COMPASSION, CONSIDERATION, COLLABORATION, COMMITMENT, CALMNESS, CREATIVITY, and COURAGE. We worked on this project with love and fun because we've been both student nurses and nursing teachers. We know the scope of your undertaking.

Sylvia Rayfield
Loretta Manning

What we ARE communicates
far more eloquently than anything
we can say or do.

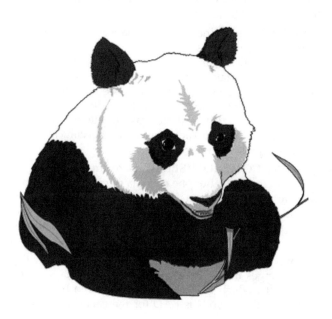

MANAGEMENT

PRIORITIZING

We want to introduce you to "MERRY MANAGER." She will be the nurse manager that will accompany you on your journey through out these first two chapters. As you can see by looking at her, she is positive both in her management style as well as in her thinking. She is outcome oriented and always attempts to understand the concerns of her nursing staff. "MERRY" is indeed one of those eagles that every nurse wants to emulate. Join us as we begin our journey through this "INSANELY EASY" and FUN book. Thank you for selecting this book for your journey! Let's get started with prioritizing nursing care.

Nurses must be able to make decisions regarding how to prioritize nursing care. Nurses are daily faced with the challenge regarding which client should be assessed (FIRST).

F FIND HYPOXIA–When the nurse has several clients to provide care for, oxygenation is always an immediate concern. Hypoxia may be a result of cardiac or respiratory complications. Physiological changes such as vital signs, skin color, or capillary refill are a few of the assessments the nurse would anticipate. Another assessment the nurse may anticipate may be an increase in anxiety or confusion. When there was no alteration in sensorium prior to the current medical condition, this clinical change may strongly represent hypoxia!

I IMMUNOCOMPROMISED–If there are 4 clients, none of which are hypoxic, but one client is receiving chemotherapy or is immunocompromised from another medication or medical condition, then this client should be evaluated first. The objective is to prevent infections from being transferred to the client.

R REAL BLEEDING–A client that is hemorrhaging from a trauma, surgery, etc. is also a priority. This client will present with changes in the vital signs, skin color, temperature, urine output, etc. which will result in alteration in tissue and organ perfusion. BLEEDING is BAD for the client! Let's get on with the care!

S SAFETY–Any client who is at risk for injury from increased intracranial pressure or confusion from delirium or dementia would be important to assess first. A toddler playing with a balloon would also be at risk for injury.

T TRY INFECTION–If a client is septic with a high fever, and has an order for blood cultures and antibiotics, this client may be the priority to assess first. The priority for this client is to obtain blood cultures as ordered prior to starting the antibiotic therapy.

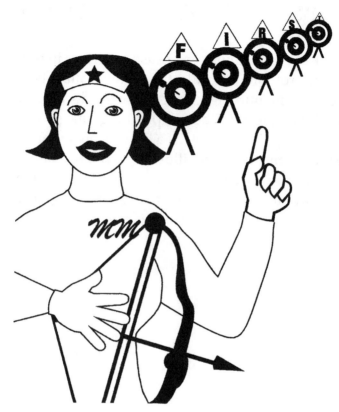

©2002 I CAN Publishing, Inc.

MERRY MANAGER is our STAR manager, because she has the qualities that we believe are so important in any manager.

S STRENGTH to grow, help and allow others to grow

T THE "HAPPINESS FACTOR" (comfortable in her own shoes, is not a victim and does not blame)

A A VISIONARY that can think "out of the box"

R REACTIVE LAST, proactive first

PROPER IDENTIFICATION

One of the number one causes of errors in hospitals is inappropriate identification. Nurses must be meticulous in identifying clients prior to documentation, administering medications, planning care, procedures, and report. For example, if a client is out of touch with reality from a delusion, illusion, or hallucination, then the priority of care prior to administering medications would be to properly identify the client to assure safety. Safety is ALWAYS a priority of care!

PROPER IDENTIFICATION

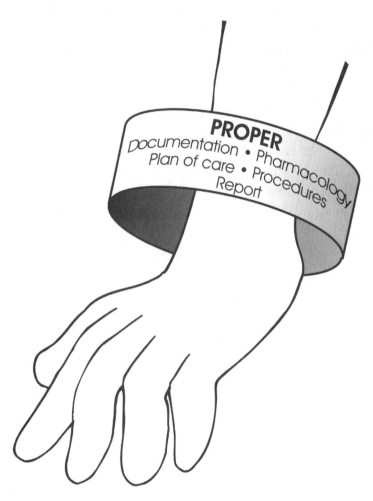

HIPAA

The Hippo looking around the privacy fence will assist you to remember the most common standards utilized by nurses to comply with the HEALTH INSURANCE PORTABILITY AND ACCOUNT-ABILITY ACT (HIPAA). While not all inclusive, the reminders on the next page affect hospitals, physicians and other provider offices, pharmacies, and many other entities that are privy to private information. These entities must, according to federal law, implement standards to protect and guard against the misuse of individually identifiable health information. Compliance with HIPAA standards allows nurses to provide care within the legal scope of practice.

HIPAA

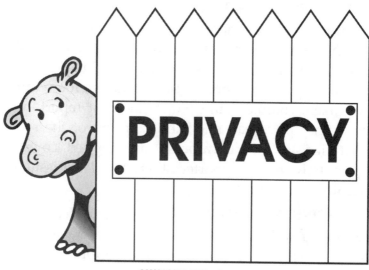

©2008 I CAN Publishing, Inc.

H ow to release information to health care workers that "need to know"

I mpermissible uses and disclosures result in lawsuits

P rotect privacy of individually identifiable health information

A rrange for sharing information with families in a discreet manner

A ccess by clients to medical records including the right to see and copy

LEGAL ASPECTS

DUE PROCESS–Hospitals, nursing homes, and other institutions where nurses practice have policies and procedures. For example, the little old lady climbs over her bedrail and falls on the floor. Due process is to pick her up, take her to x-ray, evaluate if anything is broken, complete and file an incident report, and notify her physician and family. If any of the steps identified as "the due process" are skipped, covered up, not charted or reported, there is a legal issue of negative proportions.

DECISION/ARBITRARY–The nurse's decision to refuse a family member visiting rights because she doesn't like their pierced nose and motorcycle jacket may be arbitrary and cause a legal issue.

DEPRIVATION OF PROPERTY–Nursing faculty that choose to give course outlines to all students during the first day of class, but refuse to share with the student who shows up the next day may be dealing with "deprivation of property".

DEPRIVATION OF CONFIDENTIALITY–The nurse that discusses one client with another may be dealing with a **deprivation of confidence**.

INTEGRITY TAKES US A LONG WAY
IN KEEPING US OUT OF COURT!

LEGAL ASPECTS

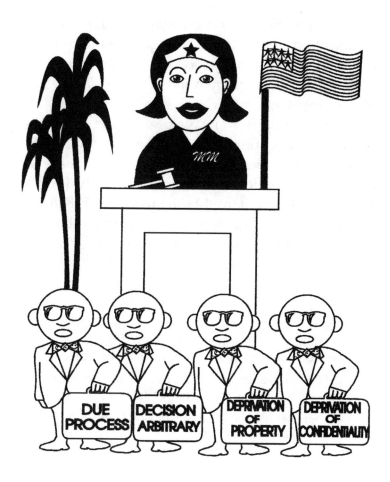

DELEGATION

The "DELEGATOR" delegates tasks but NOT responsibility. He tells his colleague how to be helpful to him. *(It is important to practice excellent communication skills or the colleague may become "stinky" like a skunk!)* Management issues are a part of the NCLEX® Test Plan. Delegating has always been a part of management, but the scope of practice laws vary from state to state regarding the meaning of delegation. These facts are a generalization and should generally keep the DELEGATOR out of trouble on the NCLEX®. Before we **TELL** someone to do something we know that we're usually legally responsible for the outcomes. These are the facts we need to know.

T **TAUGHT**–Has the individual been taught the skill, treatment or service?

E **EVALUATE**–Just because they have been taught how to do something doesn't mean they are competent to do it. Has their return demonstration been performed and documented?

L **LICENSE**–Does the individual have or need a license to do this task? Is it within their scope of practice?

L **LISTS**–What lists of standards of care (agency policies) are written regarding this task?

Remember–The DELEGATOR delegates the task
NOT THE RESPONSIBILITY!

DELEGATOR

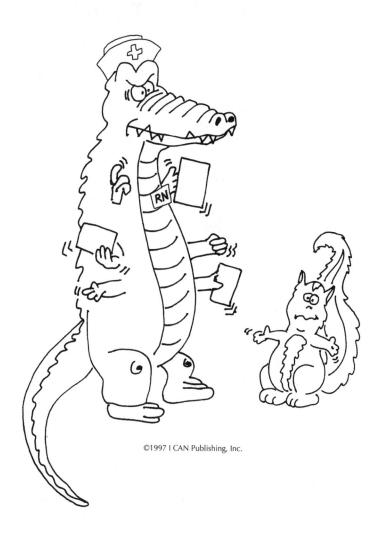

ANCILLARY PERSONNEL LIMITATIONS

LPNs and UAPs are key players in the current health care team. In order to delegate appropriately, the RN must be aware of their scope of practice. Since it will take more space than we have to review what both of these groups can do, let's review the **PART** of care the LPNs cannot do and the UAPs **CAN'T** do. This is based on our interpretations of the various Nurse Practice Acts as reflected across the United States of America.

LPN

P PLAN IN ISOLATION OF RN–LPNs plan in collaboration with the RN. They will not do this in isolation of the RN. **PUSH IV MEDICATIONS**–The current LPN standard is not to push IV medications.

A ASSESS INITIALLY–LPNs will participate in ongoing assessments; however, the RN is responsible for the initial assessment. **ANALYZE**–LPNs do not make nursing diagnosis or analyze the nursing care.

R REVIEW-EVALUATE IN ISOLATION OF RN–The LPN is responsible for collaborating with the RN during the evaluation process.

T TEACH INITIALLY–While LPNs may be involved in the teaching process, they are not responsible for initiating the teaching process. This is the responsibility of the RN. The LPN may reinforce teaching.

UAP

C CAN'T IRRIGATE A FOLEY–The UAP should not conduct this intervention. **CAN'T MAKE CLINICAL DECISIONS**–UAPs can make observations, but are not responsible for clinical decisions.

A ANTICIPATE CLINICAL CHANGES–UAPs should never be accountable for anticipating client's clinical changes.

N NO INVASIVE PROCEDURES–UAPs should not be accountable for any invasive procedures or specialized procedures.

T TEACH–UAPs are not responsible for teaching.

ANCILLARY PERSONNEL LIMITATIONS

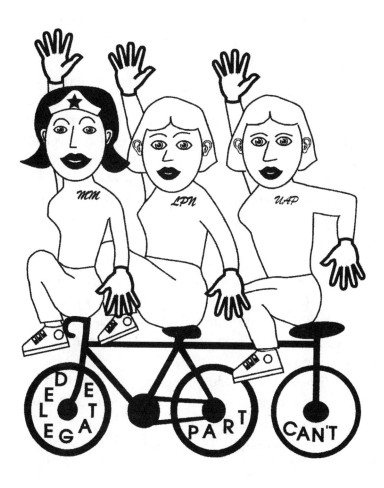

TASKS TO BE DELEGATED TO THE UAP

"**BART**" (on the next page) will assist you in remembering what tasks can be delegated to the UAP (Unlicensed Assistive Personnel).

"**BART**" will assist you in also remembering that UAPs are a link to the strength and success of any nursing team. Nurses need to remember that nursing consists of many tasks that require critical decision-making, so this must be considered when delegating tasks to the UAP. For example, it is acceptable for the UAP to **bathe** a client; however, if the client is in acute distress or has any complications such as a decubitus ulcer, then the nurse may implement the bath due to the need for ongoing clinical assessments.

Ambulation that is routine can also be delegated to the UAP. Of course, if there are any complications, such as with hypotension, syncope, and/or post-op implications, then the nurse must be present for this intervention.

Routine tasks that do not require **critical thinking** such as obtaining a urine specimen, stool for blood, etc. are acceptable to delegate to the UAP. It will be the nurse who will make clinical judgments and decisions based on the data.

TASKS TO BE DELEGATED TO THE UAP

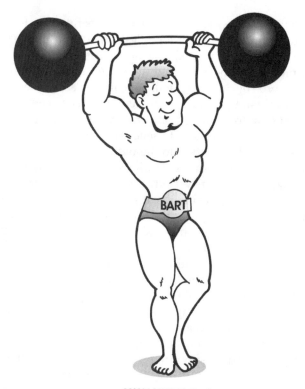

©2008 I CAN Publishing, Inc.

B aths (Routine and uncomplicated)

A mbulation

R outine tasks

T asks that do not require critical thinking

NURSES WHO FLOAT BETWEEN UNITS

The *"nurse float"* will assist you in remembering how to decide which nurse to send to a unit for a designated shift due to shortages in staffing. When making a decision on who to send to another unit, it is important to consider the **functions** of the unit such as the type of client who will be requiring assessment, planning, and evaluating. Nursing judgment cannot be delegated. The nurse must **look** for expected outcomes with assignments which indicate that it would be safe to send a nurse to provide care for this stable client. In addition to the outcomes, it is important to evaluate the clinical condition. **Omit** delegating **specialized care** to nurses who float to a new unit to assist when staffing is short. For example, if a medical surgical nurse floats to the Pediatric Unit, it would not be appropriate to delegate an infant who is in Bryant's traction to this nurse since this traction is specific to pediatrics. The **acuity** of the client must also be considered. The more unstable a client is with numerous medications, numerous systems involved in the medical condition, and unexpected outcomes, the less likely it will be that this is who will be delegated to the floating nurse. The **age** of the client is another consideration when delegating to a nurse coming in from another floor. The younger and older a client is, the quicker the clinical findings can change. If a medical surgical nurse is being pulled to the Pediatric unit, then the appropriate age of client for this nurse would be an older child versus a newborn or infant. This developmental stage has very specific clinical assessment findings that are unique to this group. If the nurse had not worked with this young stage of development, then it is a possibility that they may not remember the specific information. Always consider the **accountability** an issue when delegating. One of the major considerations when delegating is to make certain that the nurse has appropriate knowledge to implement the **tasks** that are delegated. It is a great idea to be knowledgeable of your institution's orientation clinical check off sheet. This will provide you with a compass to guide you in the appropriate direction when it comes to delegating to a nurse who is floating from another unit.

NURSES WHO **FLOAT**
BETWEEN UNITS

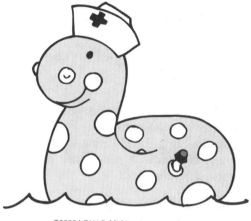

F unctions of assessment; planning, evaluating nursing judgment cannot be delegated

L ook for expected outcomes with assignments
ook at clinical condition of client

O mit specialized care

A cuity, accountability and age must be considered

T asks (knowledge required)

COST EFFECTIVENESS

"MERRY MANAGER" is responsible for managing both the quality of nursing care as well as the financial budget. It is imperative for her as well as all nurses to be cost effective. **SAVE** will assist you and "MERRY" in reviewing some strategies to achieve the outcome of cost effectiveness.

S STAFF–When making assignments, the selection of the appropriate nursing personnel is a key component in being cost effective. If an LPN is able to provide the nursing care safely and efficiently, it is not financially wise to assign the RN to the same client.

A AVOID DUPLICATION–This will also assist in providing cost effective care. For example, if a department has an unlicensed nursing personnel scheduled to run arterial blood gases to the lab, but the individual is only busy during the morning; it is wise to share this staff member with another unit and share in the cost.

V VIEW INFECTION–"AN OUNCE OF PREVENTION IS WORTH A POUND OF CURE". Infections are expensive! Wash those hands and practice universal precautions.

E EDUCATE–Discuss the budget with the nursing staff. *(An informed consumer is a smart shopper.)* AN INFORMED STAFF MEMBER CAN BE A SMART MANAGER!

COST EFFECTIVENESS

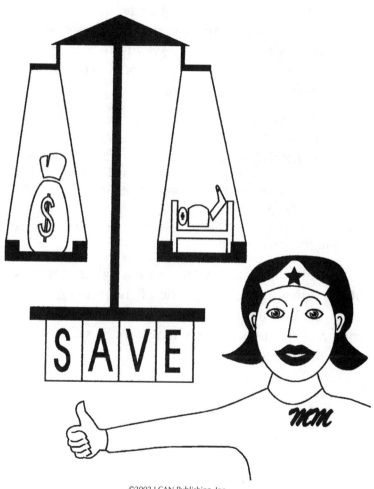

DISASTER PLAN

A disaster plan needs to be activated when there is a life threatening risk and a large number of clients must be evacuated from the hospital, assisted living units, etc. "MERRY" needs a way to remember which clients to remove first from the rooms. **ABC** will assist in organizing this information!

A AMBULATORY–The priority is to evacuate the largest volume of clients initially.

B BED RIDDEN–The bed ridden clients will be the next group to be evacuated from the rooms. Actually, the ambulatory group may be able to assist in getting this group evacuated more quickly.

C CRITICAL CARE–The last group of clients to be evacuated will be the critically ill.

The ultimate objective in a disaster plan is to evacuate volumes of clients. If the clients with numerous tubes and IVs are evacuated initially, this will slow the process down. Fewer clients will be safely rescued from the disaster.

DISASTER PLAN

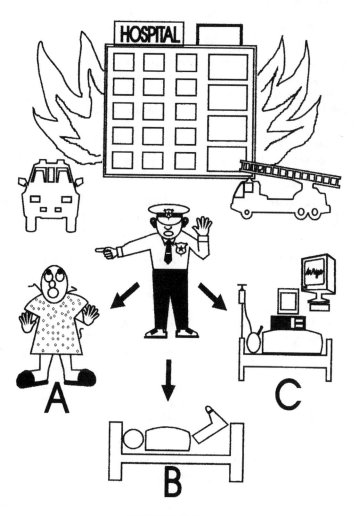

TRIAGE

Nurses are required to "**TRIAGE**" clients in the emergency department, during a disaster, or at the scene of a trauma. "**TRIAGE**" is setting priorities for care based on the client's ability to survive with adequate intervention.

Clients involved in a trauma will be evaluated initially. The priority concerns with these clients include the 4 B's (**Breathing, Bleeding, Broken Bones, Burns**). Clients experiencing hypoxia from alteration in the respiratory/cardiac system should also be triaged.

If the medical condition is chronic, however, and the client presents to the clinic for a routine visit, then this client would not be a priority.

ICP—Clients that present with head trauma, alterations in the level of consciousness, or numerous head and facial abrasions and lacerations, must be evaluated quickly.

AN INFECTION—Clients that present to the emergency department with a severe infection may proceed to go into septic shock.

GI—Clients presenting with a GI bleed must be triaged. The client may present with a history of taking NSAIDS or steroids. The client usually presents with epigastric pain characterized as being sudden, severe, and diffuse. Stools and nasogastric drainage may have blood present. The abdomen may be distended. Vital signs will change in correlation with overall condition. Clients with a very low or very high **Glucose** reading should be triaged as well.

ELIMINATION—Clients presenting with problems voiding or signs of pyelonephritis should be triaged.

Note: Remember, a client who has fixed and dilated pupils, not breathing, and no heart rate present will not be triaged!

TRIAGE

T rauma

R espiratory/cardiac

I CP

A n infection

G I, Glucose

E limination

MANAGEMENT: SAFETY

Management is currently the largest piece of the NCLEX-RN® Exam and further points can be found in the National Council of State Boards of Nursing's *Detailed Test Plan* under Safe Effective Care. We have used the word **SAFETY** as an acronym to help you remember these key concepts. Each client must have a **system specific assessment** before decisions are made regarding their care. We have placed these assessments at the beginning of each chapter. The manager is responsible for evaluating the staff and determining their skill in this area. **Accuracy of orders and assignments** will not be accurate without a client assessment.

There is such a shortage of health care workers that knowing what to do **first** is vital. The setting of **priorities** contributes to the safe effective care of the client. The shortage of health care workers has been suggested as adding to the number of medication errors that are made especially in hospitals. We must diligently **evaluate the pharmaceutical products** that we administer. Many of our clients are taking medications for many years instead of many days. For this reason, we are responsible for teaching about the interactions of their drugs, foods and alternative complimentary agents. We must also be concerned about cost control. Why administer a high cost medication if it is not going to have the desired effect?

Speaking of cost containment-infection has a devastating effect on cost. This is not just dollar cost, but cost in well-being, family dynamics, length of time to recover, and the list goes on and on. **Teach** and practice **infection control** tops the list of hospital nightmares and the NCLEX-RN® Test Plan.

Most of us know what cYa means. In this instance, we are meaning to cover your assets. The things listed under the last heading of SAFETY are the reasons for law suits. Managers are responsible for safe effective care of their clients and their staff and must be unremitting and constant in preventing these issues.

MANAGERS

S ystem-specific, focused assessment

A ccuracy of orders/assignments

F irsts—prioritize, especially in emergencies

E valuate pharmacology

T each and practice infection control

c**Y**a–cover your assets—identification, confidentiality, privacy, falls, suicide, drugs, electrical hazards, malfunctioning equipment, malfunctioning staff

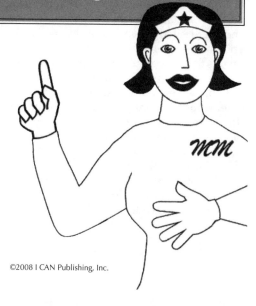

ACCURACY OF ORDERS

Just because a health care provider writes an order or gives a verbal order does not mean that we as nurses should carry out the order. We are professionals and must stand on our own two feet to determine if the order is right. We are legally responsible for our mistakes and our client if we administer the wrong medication or perform any treatment that is harmful to any person. For this reason, we must determine the accuracy of the order.

Our responsibility is to think critically and always be alert for potential errors. We want the client to receive safe care that will assist in maintaining great blood flow to our client versus reducing circulation which may reduce it to a **"DRIP."** **"DRIP"** will assist you in remembering information about *"accuracy of orders."*

For example, is the **diagnostic test** appropriate for the client? If a client had diabetes mellitus for twenty years, along with renal impairment, then any diagnostic tests ordered requiring dyes should be questioned. If a client has an order for liver biopsy, but is currently bleeding due to alteration in coagulation studies, then this order would also be questioned. With this data, the order should be contraindicated. This is why it is so very important to ALWAYS assess the client or evaluate labs prior to any intervention.

A question the nurse always has to ask, "Is this procedure **right** for the client?" When the nurse **interprets the order**, it is imperative that the questions consistently asked include: "Is this order correct for this client? Are the abbreviations correct? Is the order clear?"

Pharmacology is a top reason for alterations in client safety during hospitalization. In order to understand the accuracy of orders, nurses must understand the action of the drug, the priority in nursing care, and the desired outcomes of the medication. Nurses must have an understanding of drug-drug, food-drug interactions, and medical conditions that may result in complications from specific medications.

Our client must be able to trust us to think about every incident. Put yourself in your client's place. If you suffered from the same disease, would the ordered medication be safe for you to take? Is the dose correct? Should you receive a medication if you have had a previous allergic reaction? Should your right leg be cut off if your left leg is the one with gangrene? Should you be given a breathing treatment if you have a broken finger?

The most important gift that we can give to our client is our full attention and our brain power. Think about what you are doing! The accuracy of orders will likely determine the client's well-being. Remember—it is one thing to be a critical thinker, but the key to delivering quality, safe, client care is to have the courage to clarify and verify any orders that may be inaccurate.

ACCURACY OF ORDERS

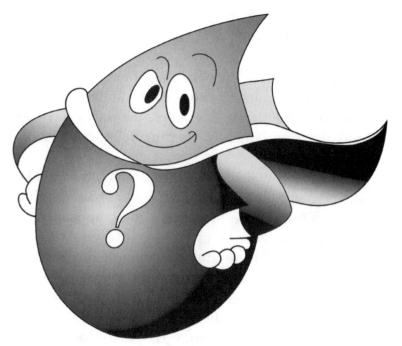

D iagnostic tests

R ight procedure

I nterpretation of order

P harmacology

COVER YOUR ASSETS (CYA)

Most of us have an idea what CYA means. For the purpose of this book, we are going to call it "COVER YOUR ASSETS"!

One of the most important assets that we have as a nurse is our nursing license. We cannot work as a nurse and take care of sick people unless we have this credential. Consequently, we must CYA to make sure we keep it.

Things that will cost our license include mistakes such as medication errors. If a client needs restraints, then it is imperative to manage these appropriately by having an order from the provider of care. It is also important for the nurse to document neurovascular checks. It is also important to document when the restraints were removed to allow for mobility and skin assessment. If a client falls, we can be sued for neglect and our license removed. Lack of confidentiality is a big problem that the nurse might be blamed for. Assigning clients to impaired staff (involved with drugs or alcohol) can turn into a crisis! Equipment that is broken and allows the client to be injured is serious trouble.

Being very present, paying attention to everything, caring, and CYA can keep us out of a "mess."

CYA

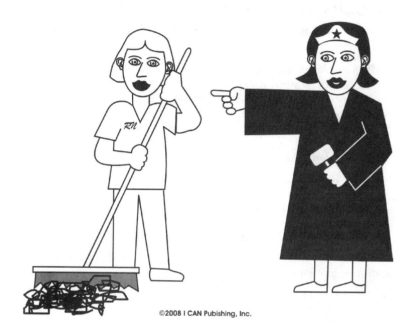

©2008 I CAN Pubishing, Inc.

M edication errors
anage restraints

E nsure confidentiality, and identity

S afe equipment (prevent falls)
afe staff

S afe delegation
uicide assessment

THE 8 RIGHTS TO MEDICATION ADMINISTRATION
(The 5 Rights plus 3 Very Important Rights to Decrease Errors)

The nurses' responsibility in safely administering medication is influenced by several major factors. These include guidelines for safe medication administration, pharmacological implications of the medication, and the legal aspects of medication administration. The "5 Rights" to medication administration are what we are going to review here.

As you can see on the next page, these "5 Rights" include:

1. Right client or Who.
2. Right drug or What.
3. Right dosage or Which.
4. Right time or When.
5. Right route of administration or Where.

We have included 3 other Rights that are imperative for safe medication administration. These include:

6. Right rationale—Why.
7. Right documentation—Write.
8. Right to know or refuse.

Nurses must not just implement the top "5 Rights", but must also understand the rationale for the client receiving the medication. If the client is receiving an antihypertensive medication and just came from dialysis with symptoms of hypovolemia, then would it be appropriate to administer this antihypertensive medication? You are so correct! Of course it would be UNSAFE! Even if you had initiated the "5 Rights", the client may develop more complications from the medication. Always understand the "WHY" prior to administering any medication!

The 7th Right is documentation—WRITE. The medication must be accurately documented on the medication record in the chart.

The 8th Right is the Right for the client to know about the medication and the Right to refuse. Clients must be taught how to safely take the med, the action of the med, and have the opportunity to refuse to take the medication. This is the right of the client!

Medication errors are a major challenge for clients in hospitals. It is imperative that we initiate these "8 Rights" in order to practice safe medication administration.

THE 8 RIGHTS TO MEDICATION ADMINISTRATION

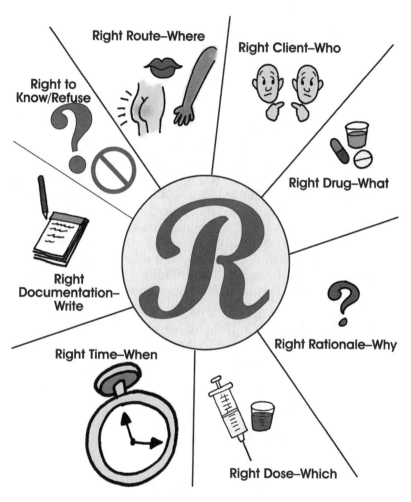

SAFETY & INFECTION CONTROL

UNIVERSAL PRECAUTIONS

Infection control is one very important nursing activity! A major problem in hospitals today is nosocomial infections. Something as simple as washing hands (**LATHERING UP**) can significantly decrease infections. Clients, family members, and health care providers must understand (**GIVE EXPLANATION**) the importance of infection control. Meticulous attention to aseptic technique when cleaning (**ORIFICES**) is effective in decreasing infections. **VERY SPECIAL HANDLING** of secretions, used equipment, needles, soiled linens, etc. is also important for decreasing infections. Nurses must remember when providing care that **EVERYONE MAY BE INFECTED**. The major concern for the nursing staff is the client who is infected and is unaware. When giving shots, starting IVs, or assisting with invasive procedures, meticulous attention must be paid to **SHARP** needles.

THE KEY TO PRACTICING UNIVERSAL PRECAUTIONS IS TO REMEMBER THE IMPORTANCE OF SAFELY HANDLING BLOOD AND BODY SECRETIONS!

In review, just remember **GLOVES** when practicing universal precautions.

G GLOVES

L LATHER UP

O ORIFICES

V VERY SPECIAL HANDLING

E EVERYONE MAY BE INFECTED

S SHARPS

GLOVES

G loves

L ather up

O rifices

V ery special handling

E veryone may be infected

S harps

G L O V E S

©2002 I CAN Publishing, Inc.

INFECTION PREVENTION: NEGATIVE PRESSURE

The sweeper is creating negative pressure, so the germs do not go out of the client's room. This is exactly the kind of pressure the client needs when there is a medical problem with tuberculosis, varicella, or the measles.

In addition to this type of pressure, the nurse needs to wear respiratory protection (masks or face shields) when entering the room. There needs to be limited transportation and client movement out of the room.

NEGATIVE PRESSURE

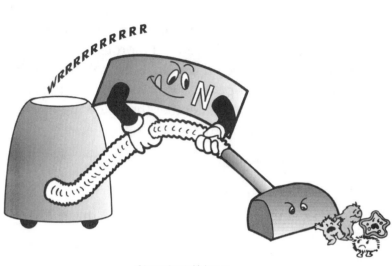

INFECTION PREVENTION: POSITIVE PRESSURE

Clients who are in neutropenic precautions or high risk for developing an infection from burns, immuno-compromised, etc. will need to be protected from any type of organism. The image illustrates this by Positive Paul attempting to push any organism out the door by positive pressure. Remember the following to assist you in understanding this concept.

Positive

Pressure

Positively

Prevents

Patient infection by

Pushing air out

POSITIVE PRESSURE

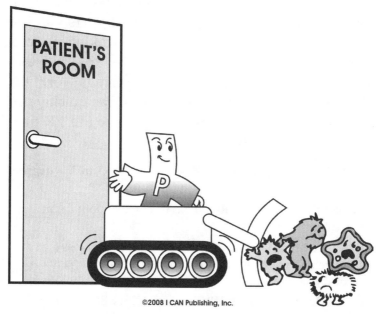

©2008 I CAN Publishing, Inc.

P ositive

P ressure

P ositively

P revents

P atient infection by

P ushing air out

FEVER

FEVER is the point where heat production exceeds heat loss. Our little digital thermometer is feeling bad. He has an ice pack on his head. His slippers indicate he is comtemplating a tepid bath. He is taking his acetaminophen or ibuprofen to prevent a rapid rise that may cause seizures. If none of these things work, the 100.4° Fahrehheit that can be tolerated can quickly rise to a dangerous level, especially at peak FEVER time late in the afternoon.

F FAHRENHEIT (97 to 100 degrees F) or (36.1 to 37.8 degrees Celsius)

E ENDOGENOUS PYROGENS reset the hypothalamic center.

V VOLUME NEEDS increase secondary to heat loss (i.e., increased metabolism, shivering, sweating, evaporation, and vasodilation).

E EVALUATE THE SOURCE VIA LABS: CBC with differential, urinalysis, blood culture, and chest x-ray. Evaluate trends in Temp. before a major problem with sepsis occurs.

R RISK FACTORS—viral or bacterial illness, environmental factors, tissue damage, biological agents, endocrine disorders

ALERT! GREATER THAN 107° F = DEATH OR IRREVERSIBLE BRAIN DAMAGE!

FEVER

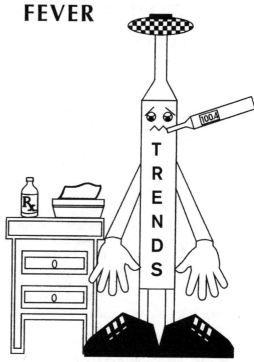

©2002 I CAN Publishing, Inc.

F ahrenheit
(97°-100° F)

E ndogenous pyrogens
Evaluate trends in Temp.
before a major problem
with sepsis occurs.

V olume needs

E valuate source via labs

R isk factors

METHICILLIN-RESISTANT STAPHYLOCOCCUS AUREUS (MRSA)

Methicillin-resistant staphylococcus aureus (MRSA) is a common drug-resistant organism found in health care facilities. MRSA is currently being treated with Tetracycline and Bactrim. **Many cultures** must be done to identify the problem. Many different infections may be a result of this pathogen such as respiratory, skin, and urinary infections. As with other organisms, the nurse is not always able to tell that the client is infected. MRSA is spread primarily by direct and indirect contact. Occasionally it is transmitted through the respiratory and urinary tracts. Standard precautions will prevent the spread of MRSA, particularly in the skin and urine infections. If the MRSA is in the wound or urine, contact precautions are used. If the MRSA is in the respiratory tract then droplet precautions are used.

When incorporating Standard Precautions, **gown, gloves, and goggles** should be worn. Gloves must be worn when touching body substances, mucous membranes, nonintact skin, and items that are contaminated. They should be changed frequently after contact with infected items and material. If soiling is likely, then gowns should be worn. If body substances are going to be splashed, then a mask/face shield is indicated. Handwashing is always important to consider. Wash hands before and after care.

If MRSA is in the respiratory tract and droplet precautions are used, then a private room is necessary. There should be 3 feet of space between the client/resident and visitors. This can create a feeling of **social isolation** for the client. If it is necessary to transport the client in the hospital, then the client must wear a mask. The linen must be bagged to prevent contamination of self, environment, or outside of bag. Infectious trash must be discarded to prevent contamination of self, environment, or outside of bag. Masks/face shield for staff and visitors must be worn for individuals who are within 3 feet of the client. Noncritical care equipment should be limited to a single client. Hands must always be washed after completion of care and all of the gowns, gloves, etc. have been removed. Standard Precautions are always adapted in addition to the other specific types of isolation.

Since MRSA is such an **active infection**, it is imperative that meticulous attention is paid to isolation techniques. Remember, infection control is one of the top activities on the NCLEX-RN®™ test plan.

MRSA

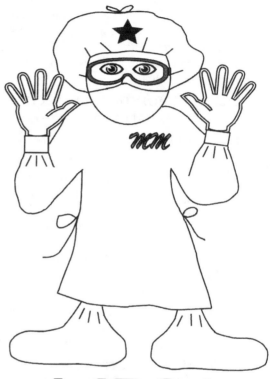

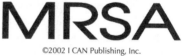

©2002 I CAN Publishing, Inc.

M any cultures

R equires gown, gloves, goggles

S ocial isolation

A ctive infection

BETA STREP

The 3 BEES help you to remember that with a B STREP infection it is wise to consider getting 3 cultures, administering 3 does of anti-infectives, and if momma BEE is pregnant she should be given her medication at the time of diagnosis as well as 2 more doses during delivery.

B BETA-HEMOLYTIC STREPTOCOCCUS–predominate causative agent in neonatal sepsis

S SCREENING–identify maternal carrier at 35-37 weeks gestation by vaginal swab

T TREATMENT–Currently if the client is found to be positive, the prophylaxis usually starts with labor, rupture of the membranes, or fever over 104° and continues until effective. CBC with differential and blood cultures are useful tests to determine this. If the infant is symptomatic, Penicillin G or other antibiotics are administered. Protocols often change for this treatment.

R RISK FACTORS–maternal GBS during pregnancy, < 37 weeks gestation, sibling with prior GBS infection, rupture of membranes > than 18 hours, intrapartum temp greater than 100.4° Fahrenheit or 38° celcius

E EVALUATE INFANT for s/s of sepsis usually appearing in first 48 hours–respiratory distress most common (apnea to mild tachypnea, labored breathing, increased oxygen requirements, mechanical ventilation), lethargy, poor feeding, hypoglycemia, temperature instability (hypothermia most common)

P PROPHYLAXIS should be given to mothers at the start of labor or when membranes rupture. If not accomplished due to precipitous delivery, treatment of the neonate should be considered.

BETA STREP

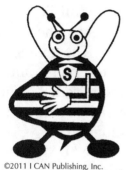

©2011 I CAN Publishing, Inc.

B eta-hemolytic streptococcus

S creening

T reatment

R isk factors

E valuate infant

P rophylaxis

CLOSTRIDIUM DIFFICILE

C. difficile is an antibiotic associated colitis that is currently the most common hospital acquired infection. The colitis, often caused by the administration of too many antibiotics, is dangerous (dehydration) and miserable. The word **"BAD"** on the next page will assist you to remember this often death producing situation.

The **"BAD"** news is that a relapse is common. The good news is that the condition is currently treated with Flagyl and Vancomycin.

CLOSTRIDIUM DIFFICILE

B acterial, hospital acquired

A ntibiotic associated
bdominal cramps

D iarrhea

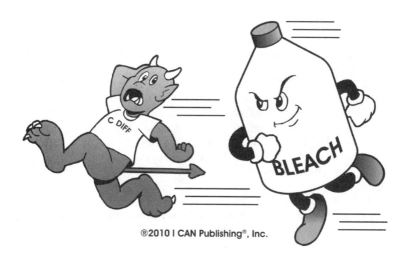

®2010 I CAN Publishing®, Inc.

Relapse is common!

ASSIGNMENT OF ROOMS

Nurses are responsible for identifying appropriate room placement for clients when they are being admitted to the hospital. The goal is decrease the **"RISK"** of complications from this process. Nurses and students have requested that we develop a technique to assist in organizing this process. **"RISK"** will assist you in organizing these placements.

If a client has internal **radiation** such as a radium implant, then the client should be placed in isolation to prevent injury to other clients. A client with an **infection** or who is immunocompromised should be placed in appropriate **isolation**. If a client has tuberculosis, varicella, or measles then airborne transmission-based precautions are important to initiate and follow. If a client has neisseria meningitis, mycoplasma pneumonia, streptococcal group A infections, or pertussis then it is important to follow droplet transmission-based precautions. Clients with easily transmitted infections by direct contact such as gastrointestinal, respiratory, skin, or wound should be placed in a private room and have contact transmission-based precautions initiated. If a client is immunocompromised (i.e., from chemotherapy, in preparation for a organ transplant, etc.), then it is important to protect the client from infections. The main point to remember is to consider infection with the selection of roommates for a client.

If a client doesn't have radiation (internal) or is not infected, then perhaps a major concern is with **safety**. Never place a combative or manic client with a depressed client or a client they could injure. If a client is at high risk for seizures due to pregnancy induced hypertension, then the client's room placement is going to be very important so there is not a lot of stimulation in the environment. Another consideration when placing clients in a room is the gender or **sex** of the client.

If none of the above issues are concerns for the client and the client is a child, then **knowing growth and development** is important to consider when placing the child with a roommate. For example, if a 6-year-old child has a fractured femur and there is another 6-year-old with a fracture or a post-op procedure with no infection, then this would be the best room placement due to the growth and developmental needs. If, however, there is another 6 year-old but the child has an infection, this would not be an appropriate roommate for the child due to the risk of transmitting the infection.

In review **"RISK"** will assist you in remembering how to select room assignments for clients.

ASSIGNMENT OF ROOMS

R adiation

I nfection/isolation

S afety, sex

K now growth and development

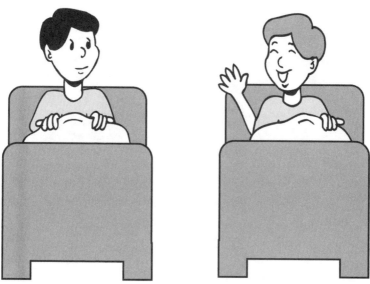

©2004 I CAN Publishing, Inc.

SAFE USE OF EQUIPMENT

Due to the number of injuries that have occurred with clients from malfunctioning equipment, it is imperative that nurses understand the importance of "**SAFE**" use.

The **System** must be without problems in order to maintain client safety.

Accident prevention can be achieved 100% of the time when the nurse evaluates **the proper functioning of the equipment PRIOR to use**. There would never be ANY client deaths from a medication due to an inappropriate bolus from the PCA pump if the nurse developed the habit of ALWAYS checking the equipment first. **Evaluating effectiveness** of the equipment is of paramount importance in providing safe care.

SAFE USE OF EQUIPMENT

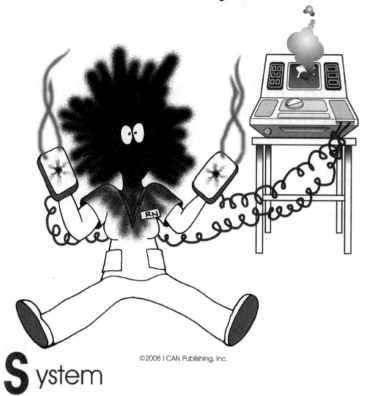

©2008 I CAN Publishing, Inc.

S ystem

A ccident prevention

F unctions properly prior to using

E valuate effectiveness

HEALTH PROMOTION

GROWTH AND DEVELOPMENT / HEALTH PROMOTION THROUGHOUT THE LIFE SPAN

From infancy to elderly there are major issues regarding health promotion that the nurse needs to review with the clients. The word SPINE will help you remember these issues.

S STRESS MANAGEMENT concerns clients throughout their lives. Children need to achieve various developmental milestones, which may be stressful during the growing process. As individuals age they must develop skill in adapting and coping to facilitate their stress management.
SAFETY is an important part of many clients' promotion of health. Safety includes anything from the toddler staying away from balloons to the elderly client watching for falls and drug/drug interactions.

P PHYSICAL ACTIVITY for the child to develop, activity to increase cardiovascular health and decrease osteoporosis are vitally important in health promotion.

I INTERPERSONAL RELATIONSHIPS are important to nurture. They prolong life and increase happiness. As the child grows into school age, their peers become increasingly more important in their life. During the working adult life, intimacy is an important developmental task.

N NUTRITION is of paramount importance throughout the lifespan to promote health and prevent disease. It is important that the adult takes in an average of 3 servings of milk, meat, vegetables, and fruits and 6 servings of bread or rice a day.

E ENVIRONMENTAL SAFETY is an important issue. We want to teach the importance of avoiding abuse, violence, poisoning, smoke inhalation, chemical spills and other noxious elements that put our life at risk.

GROWTH AND DEVELOPMENT/ HEALTH PROMOTION THROUGHOUT THE LIFE SPAN

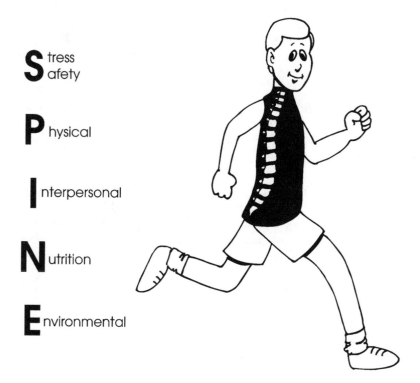

S tress
afety

P hysical

I nterpersonal

N utrition

E nvironmental

INFANCY

Check out these kids and they will help you remember milestones for these ages. Developmental task is *TRUST* versus *MISTRUST* (Erikson).

0-3 months–Recliner is in the *RECLINING* position. His head lags. At two months lifts head and chest off bed. Totally dependent. Provide toys which are soft, cuddly and colorful.

3-6 months–*SITTER*–Starts rolling over. Six months of age can SIT for short periods of time leaning forward on hands. *This age is known as the High Roller.* They can turn quickly with their heads way up off the surface. Birth weight may double at 6 months.

6-9 months–*BOUNCER OR CRAWLER*–Can pull self to a sitting position. They start bouncing so much that they bounce out and start crawling by 8–9 months. Everything goes in the mouth. Safety precautions!

9-12 months–*CRUISER OR WALKER*–Walks with help. This age loves to cruise around furniture. The birth weight may triple and length doubled (12 months). Shows stranger anxiety; clings to mother. Continues in solitary play and can entertain self for short periods of time.

INFANCY

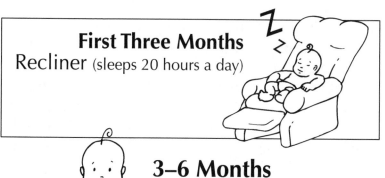

First Three Months
Recliner (sleeps 20 hours a day)

3–6 Months
Sitter with assistance,
High Roller

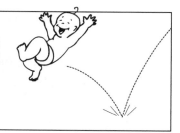

6–9 Months
Bouncer or Crawler

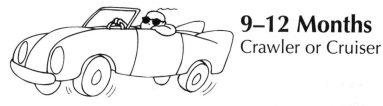

9–12 Months
Crawler or Cruiser

TODDLER (1 TO 3 YEARS)

These children are "Into everything," have temper tantrums, and are called the "Terrible Two's." The typical words used with the toddler are "NO NO." Let's think of the opposite and consider PRAISING positive behavior. Refer to image for this explanation.

Notice in the image the child has a **PUSH-PULL** toy which is a favorite. Anything that will make them mobile so they can be **AUTONOMOUS**. These children like playing side by side (**PARALLEL PLAY**), but forget sharing!

The **R** is for the eyes because at bed time if certain **RITUALS AND ROUTINES** are not continued they will not close their eyes and go to sleep. Moral of that story is consistency! **REGRESSION** may occur during hospitalization. **PRAISE** appropriate behavior and ignore the rest. (*Easier said than done!*)

The **A** is for the body because toddlers are into **AUTONOMY**. They like to help dress and undress self. **ACCIDENTS** are a leading cause of death. They may have bruises on extremities from climbing and **EXPLORING** (**E** for feet). Keep poisons out of reach.

The **I** is for the arms, so they can be comforted by their parents. Allow parents to stay with child to decrease those **S**'s (tears) from **SEPARATION ANXIETY**.

ELIMINATION (toilet training) is one of the major milestones for the toddler.

PRAISE

P ush-pull toys
arallel play

R ituals & routines
egression

A utonomy versus shame & doubt
ccidents

I nvolve parents

S eparation anxiety

E limination
xplore

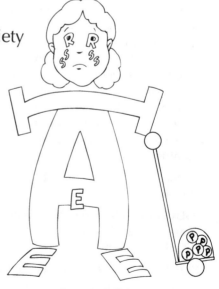

POISON CONTROL

Tommy Toxin has crawled into trouble and ingested some substance that is toxic to his body. Mom and Dad must have the poison control number available! The **national number** that will route them to the local poison control center is **800.222.1222**. If mom is in California and is visiting in Georgia using her cell phone, she will be connected to the California center. If, however, she uses a local phone and calls this national number from Georgia, she will be connected to the center in Georgia.

Currently the FDA is in dialogue regarding the current protocol for the use of Syrup of Ipecac. The current discussion is to remove this antidote from the over-the-counter medications. There is current discussion as to if it will even be available. For further update, notify the above number for current standards or the FDA.

For current practice, remember that the nurse's responsibility is to promote poison control or if poisoning does occur to prevent complications from occurring! Our initial focus for Tommy would be ABC's (airway, breathing, and circulation). "**POISON**" will assist you with Tommy's plan of care.

P PROMOTE STABILITY–Assess the condition and provide airway support, obtain IV site if necessary.

O OFF/OUT–Shower or wash **OFF** substance if it is radioactive. Remove clothing that has been contaminated, take them **OFF**! If Tommy has pills in his mouth, take them **OUT**! Eye may need to be flushed **OUT**. Antidotes may be necessary for heroin or drug overdose. Ingested substances may be taken **OUT** of the body by emesis, lavage, absorbents (activated charcoal), or cathartics. Emesis is contraindicated if a person is comatose, in shock, experiencing a seizure or has lost the gag reflex. If a low-viscosity hydrocarbon or strong corrosive (acid or alkaloid) substance has been ingested, emesis is contraindicated.

I IDENTIFY the toxic agent. Do an accurate history and identify any availabe poison.

S SUPPORT the client both physically and psychologically. Parents may feel guilty in regards to their parenting role. SUPPORT is imperative!

O ONGOING safety education regarding poison control!

N NOTIFY the poison control center, emergency facility, or provider of care for immediate care and consultation regarding treatment.

Remember the best solution to poisons
is to keep them under lock and key.

TOMMY TOXIN

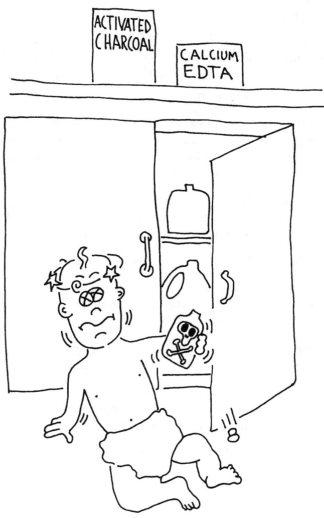

PRESCHOOL (3 TO 6 YEARS)

Preschoolers have imaginations that don't stop. The word that is characteristic of this stage is "Why?" They ask questions frequently. "Why is the sky blue?" "Why do dogs have tails?" Due to their active imagination, we have selected the word **MAGIC** to describe this stage of development.

M **MUTILATION**–They may fear mutilation. A typical statement is, "Cover my boo boo; don't let my blood run out!" Any invasive procedure is seen as mutilation (i.e., shot, I.V., enema, rectal temp., etc.).

A **ASSOCIATIVE PLAY**–They progress from parallel play to more cooperative play. An active imagination is great while pretending they are the nurse, doctor, teacher, etc.

ABANDONMENT–Children are afraid of being left.

G **GUILT**–The feeling is that if I think something bad, the thought can cause a bad event to occur. This may cause guilt for the child.

I **INITIATIVE** *versus* **GUILT**–Child is very creative and may have an imaginary companion. Imaginative toys and devices are favorites.

C **CURIOUS**–Curious about factual information regarding the environment. They always ask, "Why?"

MAGIC

Mutilation

A ssociative play
bandonment

G uilt

I nitiative
maginary playmate
magination

C urious

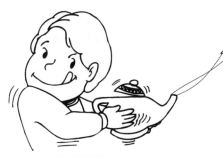

©1994 I CAN Publishing, Inc.

SCHOOL AGE (6 TO 12 YEARS)

Can you see a big dimple in the chin of this child? When you look back over your school age photo albums, what do you often see in those pictures? Many of us see those crazy little **DIMPLES**!

This will help you to associate with this group.

D   **DEATH**–The bogeyman will jump out from under the bed to get them. Be honest about funerals and burials. Encourage ventilation of thoughts and feelings.

I   **INDUSTRY** *versus* **INFERIORITY**–"Chum" period. May enjoy collecting coins, cards, etc. May enjoy sports.

     IMMUNIZATIONS should be complete before entering school.

M   **MODESTY**–More concerned with modesty and privacy. Pull those curtains and close those doors.

P   **PEERS**–The younger children play mostly with their own sex. Older child is beginning to mix with the opposite sex and learn to use the computer early. They are skilled at texting.

L   **LOSS OF CONTROL**–Hospitalization is seen as a loss of control. Allow and encourage decision making.

E   **EXPLAIN PROCEDURES**–Use terms they can understand.

DIMPLE

D eath

I ndustry versus Inferiority
mmunizations

M odesty

P eers

L oss of control

E xplanation of procedures

©1994 I CAN Publishing, Inc.

ADOLESCENT (12 TO 18 YEARS)

Adolescents are usually seen in groups or at least in **PAIRS**. Let's think about **PAIRS** while we review some milestones for the adolescent.

P **PEER** group is very important and connections are made through every social network and cell phone available. FACEBOOK and other networks allow this group to text, multitask, and collaborate in groups. Remember, carefully assess the diagnosis. Individualize the plan if client is on bed rest or in isolation.

A **ALTERED IMAGE**–They don't want to be seen as being different. Peer pressure may create problems with pregnancy, sexually transmitted diseases (STD's), substance abuse, and motor vehicle accidents. Piercings and tattoos are "IN," leaving infection as a possibility. Health Promotion programs should be developed to make adolescents aware of STD's, contraception, and the effect of drugs and alcohol on the body.

I **IDENTITY**–Adolescents may be struggling for a sense of identity. They are making important choices regarding college or career.

R **ROLE DIFFUSION**–Who are they and what are their goals? Educate families and schools regarding these struggles.

S **SEPARATION FROM PEERS**–Peer interaction may be encouraged during their hospitalization.

PAIRS

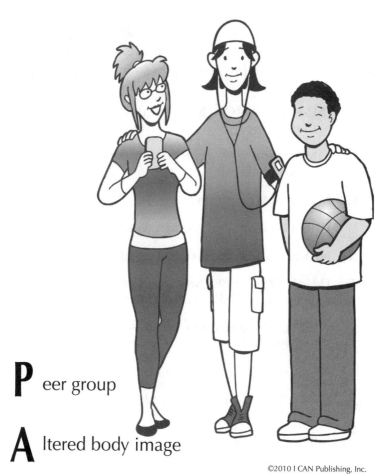

©2010 I CAN Publishing, Inc.

P eer group

A ltered body image

I dentity—Image

R ole diffusion

S eparation from peers

IMMUNIZATIONS

Those immunizations! "Nurses think they are hot shots giving us babies those shots! Let me see if there is a way that I can delay getting these immunizations!"

I   **IMMUNIZATION STATUS** (what has been given before)

M   **MMR** made with eggs–do not give with allergy to eggs or neomycin

M   **MUST** be without fever

U   **UPDATE** with new vaccines available

N   **NEVER** give in gluteals (thighs and deltoids)

I   **IMMUNE SUPPRESSION** disqualifies attenuated live vaccine, MMR, varicella, and tuberculosis

Z   **"ZEIZURE"** disorders must be controlled before administration

E   **EVALUATE** sites for local reaction

D   **DOCUMENT**–site, lot number, parental consent, and RN signature

If child is diagnosed with leukemia, HIV infection, or is receiving a high dose of steroids, wait 3 months after therapy has stopped. Measles vaccine is recommended for asymptomatic HIV-infected children.

IMMUNIZED

I mmunization status

M MR made from eggs

M ust be without fever

U pdate with new vaccines available

N ever give in gluteals

I mmune suppression disqualifies

Z eizure disorders must be controlled

E valuate sites

D ocument

DIAGNOSTIC PROCEDURES

As you review diagnostic procedures in all areas of nursing, focus on some specific areas to maintain safety for your clients before, during and after any procedure. We want to **ACT NOW** to prevent any complications with these information-gathering procedures.

A   **ALLERGIES** are an issue because many diagnostic tests use dyes. Assess for allergies, especially with iodine and shellfish which have iodine in them, prior to any procedure that uses dye. After these procedures, fluids will be encouraged to flush the dye out of the body. Some examples of procedures requiring dyes include myelograms, cardiac catheterizations, computerized axial tomography (CAT Scans), IVP's etc. *Remember the geriatric client excretes dyes slowly. Use with caution.*

C   **CONSENT FORMS** must be signed. The client should be well informed of the risks and benefits of the procedures.

T   **TEACH** the client regarding his participation and the data that the test will provide.

N   **NPO** is required for many tests. Clients and ancillary staff must be aware of this.

P **O**   **SITION** is important during and after many procedures. This information should be part of the pretest education.

W   **WHAT ARE THE VITAL SIGNS?** –VS's are an excellent way to determine the client's reaction to a procedure, especially if dye has been used.

DIAGNOSTIC PROCEDURES

A llergies

C onsent

T each

N P O

p**O** sition

W hat are the vital signs?

DIAGNOSTIC TESTING

On the previous page, we discussed a method to assist you in organizing the general concepts for diagnostic testing. Now "**DIAGNOSE**," will share some common diagnostic tests and outline some priorities for these **diagnostic tests**. "Sure Look" Holmes is taking a look in the hippo's mouth to assure he's safe! (next page) Just as "Sure Look" Holmes, the nurse is not responsible for ordering these tests, but to maintain client SAFETY before, during and after these tests.

Invasive Monitoring could represent an Intracranial Pressure Monitor (ICP), Pulmonary artery pressure reading (Swan-Ganz), or Central Venous Pressure (CVP) catheter. Some of the priority nursing considerations that may be a concern while the client has invasive monitoring include: infection, potential air emboli, patency of the line, appropriate placement of the transducer in order to assess accurately, and/or accurate interpretation of the pressure reading. If an OB client is experiencing potential complications and mandates an **amniocentesis**, then the nurse needs to be on the alert for potential risk for hemorrhaging, ongoing leaking membranes after the procedure that can result in infection, or mild discomfort at the needle site.

Gastric Diagnostic (Stool Specimen) – Some priority nursing considerations for this process may include collecting specimens in appropriate sterile container if examining for pathological organisms. Prior to the test, the client may be on a specific diet such as no red meat, beets, or food that may cause the stool to turn red which would result in a false-positive reading. The specimen must be obtained from various areas of the stool. When the paper turns blue, guaiac testing for occult blood is positive.

Nonstress Test is done to observe the response of fetal rate to the stress of activity. Client may be in a semi-Fowler's position; the external monitor is applied to document fetal activity; mother activates the "mark button" on the electronic fetal monitor when she feels fetal movement. If there is no fetal movement, the abdomen may be gently rubbed or palpated to stimulate movement; or the client may be asked to eat a light meal since blood glucose increases fetal activity. Any deceleration during the procedure must be reported to the physician.

Oxytocin Challenge Test (OCT) – Be on the outlook for late decelerations during this test. This test is all about evaluating potential hypoxia to the fetus. If the reading shows late decelerations with at least two of the three contractions, this may indicate the possibility of insufficient placental respiratory reserve. This may indicate fetal hypoxia!

Spinal (Lumbar Puncture) – Some immediate priorities prior to the procedures are to have client empty bladder and to assist in positioning so client remains immobilized during the procedure to prevent injury (lateral recumbent with knees flexed). Post-test-position client supine for at least 3 hours and sometimes up to 12 hours, to decrease occurrence of headache. Encourage high fluid intake. Observe for spinal leak from puncture site; if leakage occurs, it may precipitate a severe headache.

Electroencephalography (EEG) – Client education needs to include that there is no danger of electrical shock during the test. Evaluate if client is taking tranquilizers and sedatives since they may alter the results of test. Frequently, coffee, tea, and cola are also withheld prior to the exam. Hair should be clean prior to test; after test, assist client to wash electrode paste out of hair.

DIAGNOSTIC TESTING

D iagnostic testing

I nvasive monitoring

A mniocentesis

G astric diagnostic (stool specimen)

N onstress test

O xytocin Challenge Test (OCT)

S pinal lumbar puncture

E EG

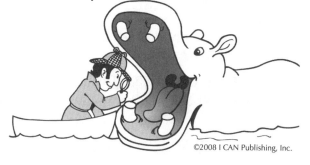

©2008 I CAN Publishing, Inc.

DANGER SIGNS IN PREGNANCY

Visualize in your mind a pregnant woman who is experiencing some complications in her pregnancy. The letters **ABC'S** will help you remember these complications.

A   **ABDOMINAL PAIN**–Abdominal pain (epigastric area) may be due to edema of the liver capsule and may indicate a convulsion is impending. A rigid, board-like abdomen during the last trimester usually indicates abruptio placenta.

B   **BLURRED VISION**–Visual disturbances may indicate hypertension elevated.

   BLOOD PRESSURE ELEVATION is a complication with severe preeclampsia.

   BLEEDING–Early bleeding could indicate a miscarriage, abortion, ectopic pregnancy or hydatiform mole. Bleeding in the last trimester may be indicative of placenta previa or abruptio placenta.

C   **CHILLS AND FEVER**–Indicative of an infection, and is never normal during pregnancy.

   CEREBRAL DISTURBANCES–Headaches during pregnancy can indicate severe preeclampsia.

S   **SWELLING**–Edema especially in the periorbital and digital areas is indicative of mild preeclampsia. Watch for **SUDDEN ESCAPE OF FLUID** (rupture of membranes)!

ABC's OF DANGER SIGNS IN PREGNANCY

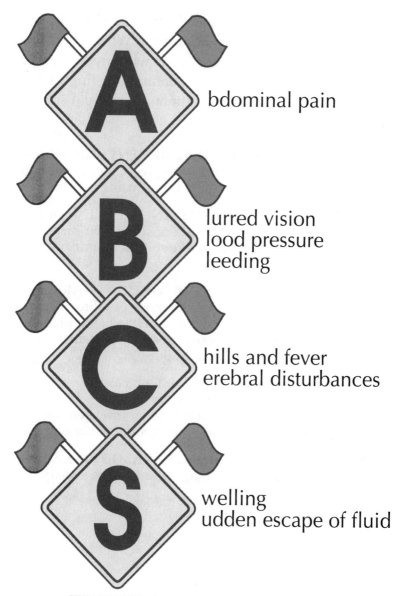

bdominal pain

lurred vision
lood pressure
leeding

hills and fever
erebral disturbances

welling
udden escape of fluid

PREGNANCY-INDUCED HYPERTENSION

This condition is specifically associated with pregnancy, preeclampsia and eclampsia. When you think about the priority nursing care with this disorder, think about **PEACE**. It is of paramount importance to provide a peaceful environment to prevent seizure activity.

P **PROMOTE BEDREST, QUIET ENVIRONMENT–** These are crucial. In severe preeclampsia, absolute bedrest and sedatives (Valium) are important.

E **ENSURE HIGH PROTEIN INTAKE** – Due to proteinuria, protein intake should be increased in the diet. Sodium intake should remain normal. Avoid diuretics.

A **ANTIHYPERTENSIVE DRUG** – (Aldomet) methyldopa widely considered first line in pregnancy may be used to decrease the blood pressure. It's safe since it doesn't cross the placental membrane. Check maternal BP, pulse and FHR.

C **CONVULSION** – Prevent or control seizures. Administer IV Magnesium Sulfate. Have the antidote, calcium gluconate at the bedside for emergencies. Decrease the environmental stimuli.

E **EVALUATE PHYSICAL PARAMETER–**Evaluate for complications of magnesium sulfate toxicity.

PEACE

P romote bedrest, quiet environment

E nsure high protein intake (1g/kg/day)

A ntihpertensive drug: (Aldomet) methyldopa, widely considered first line in pregnancy

C onvulsions (Magnesium Sulfate)

E valuate physical parameters
    1. Blood pressure
    2. Urine output
    3. Respirations
    4. Patella reflex

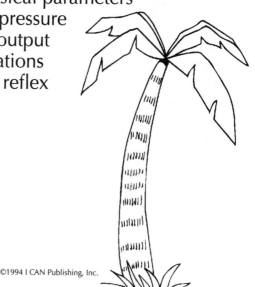

MAGNESIUM SULFATE TOXICITY

Magnesium Sulfate is the drug given to women to prevent seizures with the complication of pregnancy-induced hypertension (PIH). This medicine is a central nervous system depressant. The antidote is calcium gluconate. How can you remember the signs of too much of this medicine? Just remember that before a client has a seizure they may let out a loud **BURP**! (Do they do this in reality? Not usually; it is only a memory technique.)

Let me introduce you to Bonnie Burp. She has the following problems:

B   **BLOOD PRESSURE DECREASED**

U   **URINE OUTPUT DECREASED**

R   **RESPIRATIONS DECREASED**

P   **PATELLA REFLEX ABSENT**

Bonnie is predisposed to these side effects because magnesium sulfate is a central nervous system depressant. It acts by blocking the neuromuscular transmission.

Warning: Magnesium Sulfate cannot be used with some anesthetics as it paralyzes the client without sedation. In this situation, we must keep the client sedated.

MAGNESIUM SULFATE TOXICITY

B lood pressure decreased

U rine output decreased

R espirations < 12

P atella reflex absent

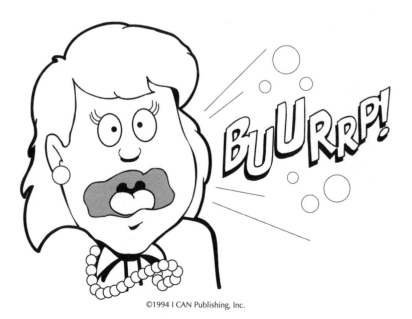

FETAL HEART DECELERATIONS: EARLY DECELERATIONS

What is happening? As you can see on the next page, there is pressure on the head of the fetus. The difference in this **EARLY DECELERATION** in contrast to a **LATE DECELERATION** is that the onset, fall and recovery of the heart rate coincide with the onset, peak and end of the contraction. This does not indicate a problem and usually occurs during the active phase of labor.

EARLY DECELERATIONS: HEAD COMPRESSION

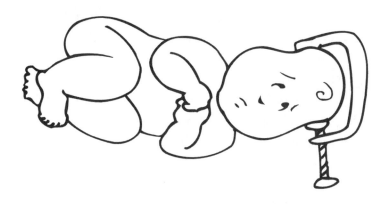

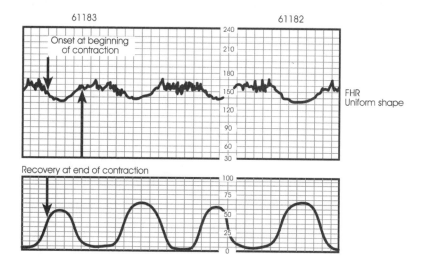

FETAL HEART DECELERATIONS: VARIABLE DECELERATIONS

VARIABLE DECELERATIONS are usually shaped like a V or a squared U. These may occur any time during the contraction cycle or may be nonrepetitive. The pathophysiology is cord compression. The nursing care is to change the position of the mother. If it lasts more than one minute, attempt upward displacement of presenting part. Mother may be placed in the knee-chest position or Trendelenburg position. This pattern may indicate a prolapsed cord. If this is the case, prepare for immediate delivery. To assist with fetal oxygenation, the nurse may give the mother oxygen.

VARIABLE DECELERATIONS: CORD COMPRESSION

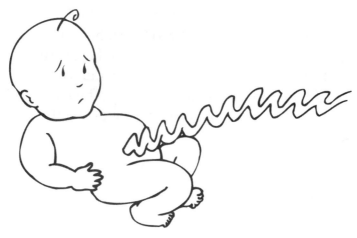

61180

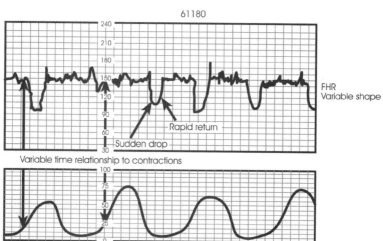

FHR
Variable shape

Rapid return

Sudden drop

Variable time relationship to contractions

FETAL HEART DECELERATIONS: LATE DECELERATIONS

LATE DECELERATIONS look similar to early decelerations but are offset to the right. They begin at about the peak of the contraction, and the nadir occurs well after the peak of the contraction. The cause of these is uteroplacental insufficiency. The focus will be on the nursing care on the pages following the rhythm strip.

LATE DECELERATIONS: UTEROPLACENTAL INSUFFICIENCY

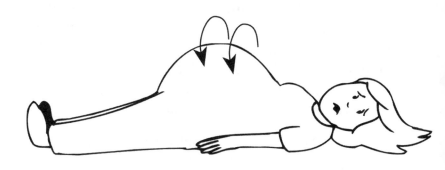

61183

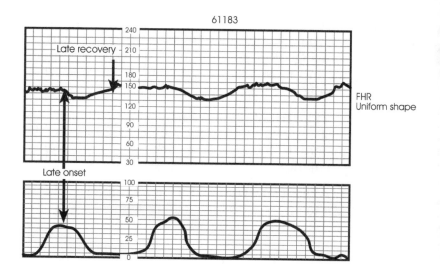

LATE DECELERATIONS

The Fire Department has come to the rescue of **FETAL DISTRESS**, and is planning to put out the problem. First, however, they must **UNCOIL** the fire hose. What does a late deceleration look like and what does it mean? It is a uniform shaped dip. The onset coincides with the peak of the contraction with the recovery occurring at the end or after the end of the contraction. It indicates uteroplacental insufficiency. If the fire department does not do something soon, the fetus is going to get into severe distress.

C **CHANGE POSITION**–Place mother in the left lateral position. For supine hypotension, change the maternal position.

O **OXYGEN**–Administer oxygen to mother to correct the uteroplacental insufficiency. If **OXYTOCIN** is infusing, stop the infusion. This may be causing uterine hyperactivity resulting in uteroplacental insufficiency.

I **IV FLUIDS**–Epidurals may cause dilation. Increasing hydration with IV fluids will increase the maternal blood pressure and the uteroplacental circulation.

L **LOWER THE HEAD OF THE BED** and elevate the feet to increase perfusion to the uterus.

LATE DECELERATIONS

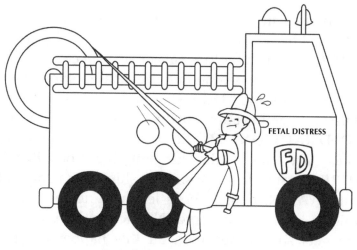

Reprinted with permission ©1994 Martha Eakes

U

N

C hange position (left side)

O xygen
xytocin—off

I V fluids

L ower head

PITOCIN

Pitty Pitocin, this pregnant woman, is slow to begin active labor, so the Doc decides to induce by using **PITOCIN**. Watch for those major side effects!

Visualize Pitty sitting in a row boat looking into a **PIT** watching the "TETANIC" sink into the "ocean" (**OCIN**). Complications of this drug are **TETANIC CONTRACTIONS**. Pitocin of course is a stimulant; so as Pitty watches the ship sink, her blood **PRESSURE** elevates! Just as a sinking ship takes in all that salty WATER, poor Pitty is left holding the excess fluid in her body (observe **INTAKE** and **OUTPUT**). She gets so nervous with all this happening that she goes into **CARDIAC ARRHYTHMIAS** causing Pitty's baby **OXYGEN** hunger and **FETAL HEART IRREGULARITIES**. This is so upsetting to Pitty that she gets **NAUSEATED** and **VOMITS** all over the row boat.

STOP THAT PITOCIN DRIP!!!!

SIDE EFFECTS OF OXYTOCIN (PITOCIN)

P ressure is elevated

I ntake and output

T etanic contractions

O xygen decrease in fetus

C ardiac arrhythmia

I rregularity in fetal heart rate

N ausea and vomiting

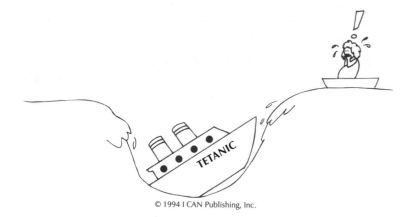

REGIONAL ANESTHESIA

Regional anesthesia is used to anesthetize one **REGION** of the body; the client may remain awake and alert throughout the procedure. The image used will assist in recalling nursing care for the different **REGIONS** of the body.

R **RESPIRATORY PARALYSIS**–Have ventilatory support equipment available. Avoid the extreme Trendelenburg position before level of anesthesia is set.

E **ELIMINATION**–Evaluate the bladder for distention. When the epidural is done on a pregnant woman, labor may be delayed due to bladder distention.

G **GASTROINTESTINAL**–Check when client last ate. Position to prevent aspiration. Antiemetics need to be available along with suction equipment.

I **INFORM OF PROCEDURE**–Does the client understand the procedure? Check for drug allergies, make sure legal permit is signed and have client empty bladder.

O **OBSERVE FOR HYPOTENSION**–Report B/P less than 100 systolic, or any significant decrease. Change client's position, administer oxygen and increase IV rate if client is not prone to CHF.

N **NO TRAUMA TO EXTREMITIES**–Support extremities during movement. Remove legs from stirrups together.

ANESTHESIA

R espiratory paralysis

E limination

G I

I nform of procedure

O bserve for hypotension

N o trauma to the extremities

©1994 I CAN Publishing, Inc.

POSTPARTUM ASSESSMENT

If a parent's newborn is a daughter, they must "BUBBLE HER" during and after feedings. This will assist you with reviewing the postpartum assessment.

B   **BREAST**–Assess for and prevent mastitis. Teach how to cleanse breasts and nipples. Support with breast feeding.

U   **UTERUS**–Fundus should be firm and in the midline. Immediately after delivery, the top of the fundus is several finger breadths above the umbilicus. The fundus then descends into the pelvis approximately one finger breadth per day. Massage the fundus if it is boggy.

B   **BLADDER**–Observe for bladder distention; it may displace the uterus. Diuresis occurs during the first two postpartal days. Evaluate for UTI.

B   **BOWEL**–Stool softeners or laxatives may be necessary. By second or third day post delivery, normal bowel movements should occur.

L   **LOCHIA**–Should not have foul odor. Rubra (dark red first 3 days), serosa (pinkish, sero-sanguinous 3 -10 days) and alba (creamy or yellowish after 10th day and may last a week or two).

E   **EPISIOTOMY**–Observe for infection and healing.

H   **HOMAN'S SIGN**– Observe for thrombophlebitis.

E   **EMOTIONAL**–Support is a must!

R   **RHOGAM** is a blood product administered at 28 weeks, and within 72 hours after delivery.

POSTPARTUM ASSESSMENT

B reast

U terus

B ladder

B owel

L ochia

E pisiotomy

H oman's sign

E motional

R hogam

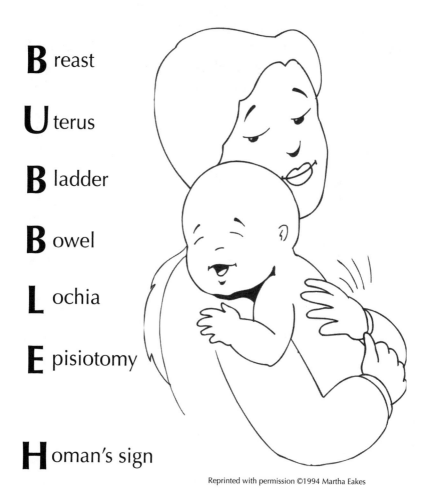

Reprinted with permission ©1994 Martha Eakes

FOODS HIGH IN FOLIC ACID

Several conditions require a client to eat a diet high in folic acid. Some examples of these are: iron deficiency anemia, chronic alcohoism, pregnancy and malnutritional anemia. Here is a visual to help you remember those foods high in Folic Acid.

FOLIC ACID

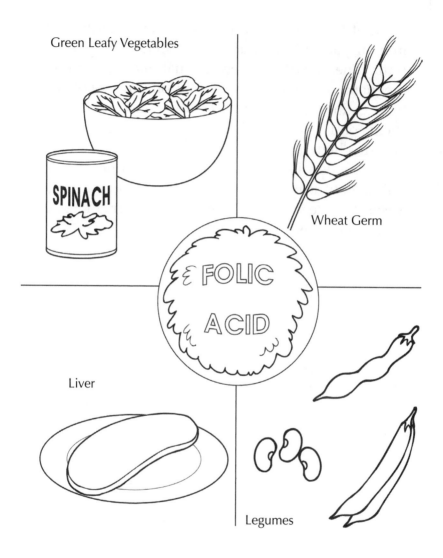

Green Leafy Vegetables

SPINACH

Wheat Germ

FOLIC ACID

Liver

Legumes

FOODS HIGH IN IRON

What type of clients need to be on a diet high in iron? If you indicated any of the following, you are right. Clients with hemodilutional anemia who are pregnant, poor dietary intake of iron, surgery of gastrointestinal tract, problems with absorption and clients on IV therapy for 10 days or more need to be on a diet high in iron.

The foods which are high in iron are: organ meats (think about an organ that plays music), red meats, fish, green leafy vegetables, raisins (the California Raisin), sunflower seeds and legumes.

IRON

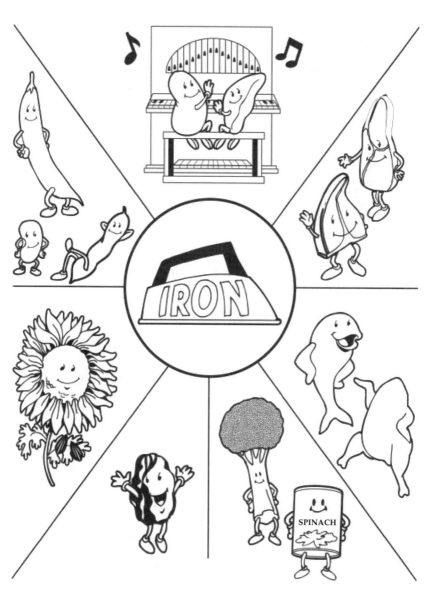

FOODS HIGH IN PROTEIN

Foods high in protein can easily be remembered if you recall the jingle *Happy To Consume My Calories Sanely*. **H**amburger, **T**una, **C**hicken, **M**ilk, **C**ottage Cheese and **S**oy Beans are high in protein.

PROTEIN

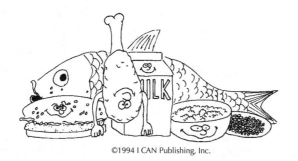

©1994 I CAN Publishing, Inc.

Happy	=	**H**amburger
To	=	**T**una
Consume	=	**C**hicken
My	=	**M**ilk
Calories	=	**C**ottage Cheese
Sanely	=	**S**oy Beans

FOODS HIGH IN POTASSIUM

An easy way to remember foods high in Potassium (K+) is the **ABC Fruit** and **Veggie Plate**. Apples, Bananas, Cantaloupe (melons) and Citrus such as orange juice are high in K+. Asparagus, Broccoli and Carrots are also high in potassium. Another vegetable to remember that is high in potassium is the potato! Teach clients about the **ABC Fruit** and **Veggie Plate**, especially those clients who are taking diuretics.

Clients with severe burns, others who have hypersecretion of the adrenal cortex or on long term steroid therapy will benefit from these foods.

K FOODS =
ABC FRUIT/VEGGIE PLATE

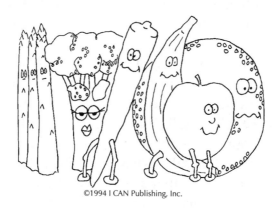

©1994 I CAN Publishing, Inc.

FRUITS	**VEGGIES**
Apples	**A**sparagus
Bananas	**B**roccoli
Cantaloupe	**C**arrots

FOODS HIGH IN SODIUM

The all-American **HOT DOG**–your way to remember foods that are high in salt (sodium). What is the first thing you must have for a hot dog? A wiener of course. Can't have a hot dog without a wiener and what is a wiener? It's processed meat in a tube that is high in salt.

Now, imagine walking through the delicatessen with us, looking up and seeing all of those tubes of meat hanging from the ceiling. Pressed ham, salami, bologna–all high in salt. Next we need a bun for the wiener. Of course, we put baking soda in our bread to make it rise (soda is salt). Next, comes ketchup which is processed tomatoes that are high in salt. Some folks will mess up a perfectly good hot dog with pickles! Did you ever make pickles? You throw cucumbers into brine (salt water). Those who have to have a chili dog, open a can of chili. Canned foods are usually high in salt. Then of course some of our German friends must have sauerkraut on their dogs which is also high in salt. So, to remember those foods high in sodium, all you have to know is **HOT DOG**!

FOODS HIGH IN SODIUM

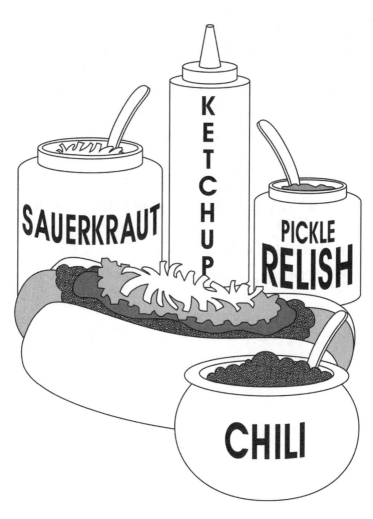

LOW RESIDUE DIET

Daddy had some sort of rectal surgery or diarrhea that makes it a necessity for him to sit on his pillow. Low residue diets are used to reduce fiber and slow bowel movements. Clients with Crohn's disease and colitis may benefit from this particular diet. Here's an easy way to remember the low residue diet.

L **LIMITED FAT AND FRIED FOODS**

O **ZERO MILK**

R **REAL FRESH FISH / UNSEASONED GROUND MEAT**

E **EGGS BOILED**, not fried

S **STRAINED FOODS**

As you can see for yourself,
this diet is NO FUN for Daddy!

LOW RESIDUE DIET

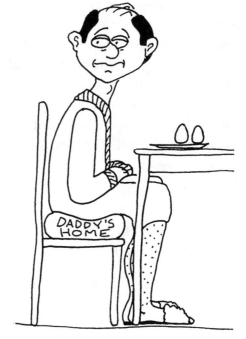

L imited fat

O zero milk

©1994 I CAN Publishing, Inc.

R eal fresh fish/ground meat

E ggs boiled

S trained foods

CELIAC DISEASE DIET

Celiac Disease is an inborn error in metabolism of barley, rye, oat products, and wheat causing malabsorption of some nutrients. Some clients who have gastritis complain of diarrhea, abdominal pain, and bloating.

This diet is known as a gluten-free diet and helps relieve the symptoms. In order to assist you to remember this diet, think of the intestinal flora like the BROW over your eye.

B	*BARLEY*
R	*RYE*
O	*OATS*
W	*WHEAT*

Remember, corn and rice may be substituted for grains in the diet.

CELIAC DIET

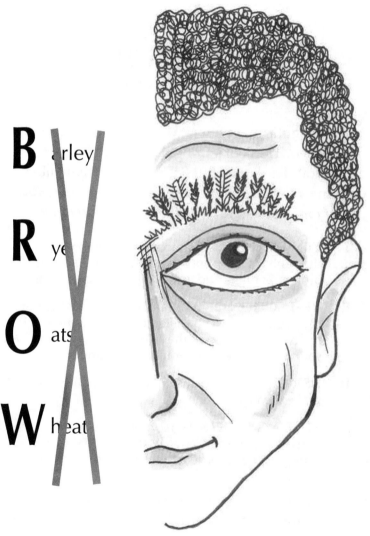

B arley

R ye

O ats

W heat

PSYCHOSOCIAL INTEGRITY

THERAPEUTIC COMMUNICATION

Therapeutic interaction takes place when **TRUST** is established. Think of joining hands with someone special to you. The letters in **TRUST** help us remember the dynamics of therapeutic communication. *Listening is one of our best assessment tools for this section.*

T **TRY EXPRESSION**–Encourage the exploration of thoughts, perceptions, feelings, and actions. Use broad openings and ask open ended questions.

R **REFLECTION OF WORDS**–Confirms to the person that you are actively listening. For example, "I am really mad at my mother for grounding me." "You sound angry because you were grounded."

U **USE OF SILENCE**–Just sit and allow the person to make the next response.

S **SETTING LIMITS**–What type of people may need to have limits set? People with personality and substance abuse disorders, affective disorders, children and spouses.

T **TIME WITH CLIENT**–Taking time with the client allows them to know that you care even if they refuse to communicate.

TRUST

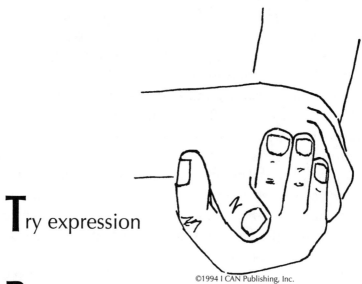

©1994 I CAN Publishing, Inc.

Try expression

Reflection of words

Use of silence

Set limits

Time with client

ANOREXIA

Anorexia is a very difficult eating disorder to overcome. The person suffering from it simply won't eat even though one coaxes and encourages. These clients are very compulsive and controlling. They strive for perfection in every facet of their life, work, school, relationships, and body. Because of their lack of subcutaneous fat, they become amenorrheic. Most anorexics are excessive exercisers, often runners. Through exercise, they burn up the few calories that they consume. Anorexics get in severe trouble when they become so malnourished that their electrolytes become unbalanced. Electrolyte imbalance, particularly hypokalemia, is a frequent cause of death in this very serious disease.

Persons with anorexia who are very thin and experiencing complications will be hospitalized until they become stable, show physiological improvement, and demonstrate weight gain. Nursing care then focuses on reversing the malnutrition, improvement in family dynamics, and individual psychotherapy. The overall goals include weight gain, development of a positive self-image, and supportive family interactions. *Weight and electrolyte balance are our best assessment tools for this issue.*

ANOREXIA

S imply won't eat

T ype A personality

A menorrhea

R un–extreme exercise

V icious cycle–lifetime

E lectrolyte imbalance;
(low–blood
hemoglobin test)

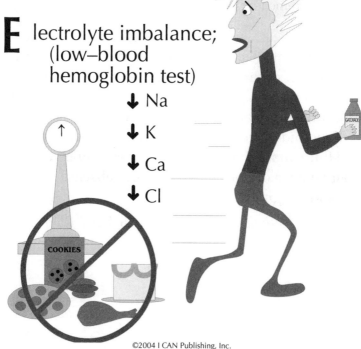

↓ Na

↓ K

↓ Ca

↓ Cl

COOKIES

BULIMIA

S **SHOVE IT IN**. Bulimics eat large amounts of food at one time. Their intake is much more than most people can imagine.

T **TOOTH ENAMEL IS DESTROYED**. Their tooth enamel becomes destroyed from gastric acid in the mouth when vomiting.

U **UPCHUCK**. Bulimics purge in a number of ways including laxative abuse and use of diuretics, but the most common is vomiting.

F **FULL WEIGHT.** Clients suffering from bulimia are usually not exceptionally thin, but maintain a normal or full weight.

F **FEAR OF FAT**. A basic issue of the disease is an extreme fear of fat.

Hospitalization for bulimia is required if complications, such as electrolyte imbalance or cardiac symptoms, occur. Nursing care is similar to that for anorexia nervosa focusing on adequate nutrition and individual and family psychotherapy.

Expected outcomes include adequate balanced food and fluid intake, healthy mucous membranes and skin, maintenance of normal weight, and absence of bingeing and purging.

Bulimics do ingest a lot of S T U F F.

BULIMIA

S hove it in

T ooth enamel is destroyed

U pchuck

F ull weight

F ear of fat

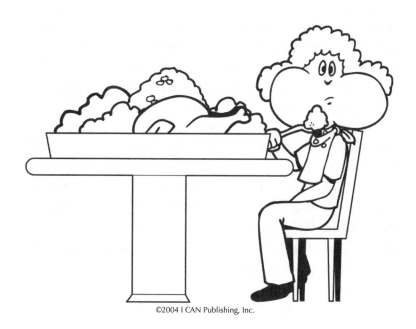

PICA

S   STUFF IS HIDDEN.

T   THINGS; i.e., hair, clay, starch. The list of non-food substances that are ingested may include clay, dirt, coffee grounds, ashes, paint chips, crayons, paper, starch, pencils, and cigarette butts.

A   ALL NON-FOOD ITEMS. The list of non-food items ingested is practically endless, but depends on availability.

S   SICK—DON'T DIGEST. Iron deficiency and impaction are the most common complications.

H   HAVE ECOLI, ILEUS.

PICA is an eating disorder characterized by the ingestion of non-food substances. It is habitual, purposeful, compulsive and most common in toddlers and pregnant women. Materials frequently eaten include clay, dirt, newspaper, laundry starch, paint chips, pencils, crayons, freezer frost, and ashes, but the list may be practically endless. Pica becomes especially problematic if the substance ingested contains a harmful ingredient, such as paint chips with lead. It also may limit the amount of nutrient rich food ingested because of feeling full. Children should be taught what is acceptable and not acceptable to eat. Pregnant women should be questioned as to any pica practices and should be helped to understand the consequences of such behavior. Iron deficiency anemia is a concern with pregnant women.

PICA

S tuff is hidden

T hings (i.e. hair, clay, starch)

A ll non-food items

S ick–won't digest

H ave ecoli, ileus

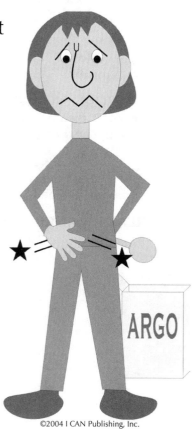

INTERVENTIONS FOR ANXIETY

ANXIETY! Welcome to nursing school! Would you agree? Perhaps we should say, "Welcome to life!" Before we can successfully help our clients deal with their anxiety, we need to remain **CALMER** ourselves.

C **CALM**–Create a comfortable, calm environment for relaxation. A quiet room with soft music may help enhance this feeling.

A **AWARENESS OF ANXIETY**– Identify and describe feelings. Modify stress producing situations.

L **LISTEN**–Listen to both client and to yourself. Implement "TRUST." Protect the defenses and coping mechanisms.

M **MEDICATIONS**–When all else fails, use those drugs. A memory tool for anti-anxiety medications is on the next page.

E **ENVIRONMENT**–Walking, crying, working and concrete tasks may help moderate anxiety. Safety is paramount if meds have to be used.

R **REASSURANCE**–Implement "TRUST."

INTERVENTIONS FOR ANXIETY

C alm

A nxiety-aware

L isten

M eds—Lexapro, Klonopin, Ativan, Xanax, Cymbalta, Buspar, and Valium

E nvironment

R eassurance

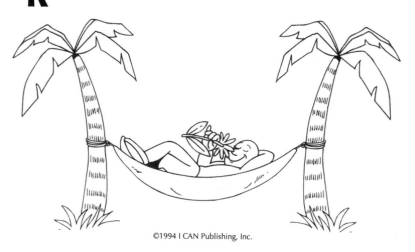

©1994 I CAN Publishing, Inc.

ANTI-ANXIETY MEDICATIONS

Clients who are anxious may feel like they are going "**BATS**." These **BATS** will assist you in remembering these anti-anxiety medications.

B   **BETA ADRENERGIC BLOCKERS** may be used for a rapid heart rate.

BENZODIAZEPINES such as alprazolam (Xanax), chlordiazepoxide (Librium), diazepam (Valium), lorazepam (Ativan) and others decrease anxiety by depressing the limbic and subcortical central nervous system.

A   **ANTIHISTAMINES** such as hydroxyzine (Atarax) may decrease anxiety if the client is a potential abuser of benzodiazepines.

T   **TRICYCLICS** and MAO inhibitors may be used for panic attacks.

S   **SSRIs** (serotonin selective reuptake inhibitors) may be effective in managing anxiety.

ANTI-ANXIETY MEDICATIONS

B eta adrenergic Blockers
enzodiazepines

A ntihistamines—COPD or potential abuse of
benzodiazepines

T ricyclics and MAO inhibitors for panic attacks

S SRIs

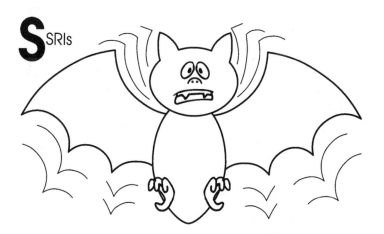

SYMPTOMS OF DEPRESSION

People that become depressed become very worried about themselves. They realize that they feel terrible and may feel trapped in these feelings. **IN SAD CAGES** will help you remember the symptoms and concerns of the depressed client.

I INTEREST is lacking in most everything. They may feel lethargic. Libido may be decreased and they are commonly apathetic. They may experience despair and become apathetic.

N NO SELF ESTEEM

S SLEEP is hard to come by. They often have several hours of sleep and then awaken with the inability of going back to sleep. Real rest is often hopeless which may add to the depression. Some people may want to sleep all the time. They are so depressed they do not want to get out of bed.

A APPETITE is very often depressed. Food doesn't look good or taste good.

D DEPRESSED people can become very tearful. They no longer smile and have a "flat affect" or no expression on their face.

C CONCENTRATION is often lacking. They may not be able to do their jobs or maintain their relationships due to the depression.

A ACTIVITY is decreased. They may become "couch potatoes" and refuse to participate in routine activities. Exercise may be an activity that they can no longer perform.

G GUILT may bring a very negative view of self, world, and future.

E ENERGY level is decreased. They may have a poverty of ideas and turn their aggressive feelings inward.

S SUICIDE precautions are mandatory. Maintaining a safe environment and negotiating a contract with them may be life saving.

SYMPTOMS OF DEPRESSION

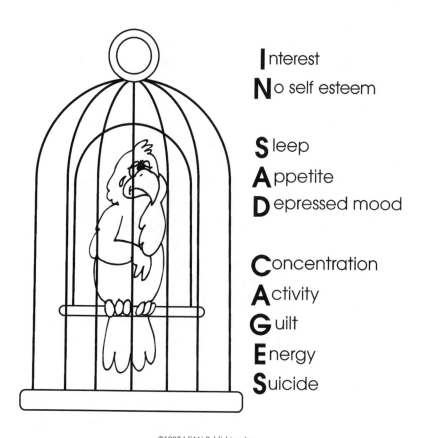

Interest
No self esteem

Sleep
Appetite
Depressed mood

Concentration
Activity
Guilt
Energy
Suicide

MANAGEMENT OF DEPRESSION

The depressed client may think of suicide. The presence of a suicidal plan, including specifics related to the method, indicates a potential risk. Harmful environment (windows in a tall building) and harmful objects (razors, knives, automobiles, etc.) should be carefully removed until the client gets in a better place. A structured environment usually works best due to their impairment in decision making.

Food may play an important role in severe depression. Some clients "stuff their feelings" and gain large amounts of weight, while others have no appetite at all and lose substantial weight. They may lose interest in food and activities surrounding their life. We can encourage participation in activities that promote a sense of accomplishment, in addition to other tasks to help increase their interest in life.

Depression, no energy, lack of self-esteem, and little concentration, often lead to decreased bathing, inappropriate attire, and decreased interpersonal friendships. Clients need friends and family at this point. We can listen, continue to establish trust, and convey a kind, pleasant concern, to help promote a sense of dignity and self-worth.

The risk for suicide is a safety issue for the client. Meticulous assessment, documentation, consultation, and necessary referrals are imperative to maintaining client safety and avoiding legal liabilities.

SUICIDE

S uicide precautions

U nusual eating

I nterest lacking, apathetic

C oncentration decreased

I nterpersonal relationships suffer

D epressed mood

E nergy/activity altered
steem depleted

ANTIDEPRESSANT MEDICATIONS—TRICYCLIC ANTIDEPRESSANTS

Tina Tricycle is sitting on the curb because she is taking new antidepressants and should not drive heavy machinery. She may need to take her medication at night so she won't be too sleepy. Notice the number 3 on her tricycle. This will remind you that it takes approximately 3 weeks for the tricyclic antidepressants to achieve a therapeutic level. Her big **HAT** will help you remember some of the undesirable effects that she may experience while on this drug.

Tina must be taught that her compliance is vital to maintain a therapeutic level. She also must know that some herbs such as St. John's Wort may cause drug/drug interactions.

Tina should not take MAO inhibitors while she is taking tricyclics. Tina wants this medicine to improve her sad face and her interest in riding her tricycle.

TINA TRICYCLE

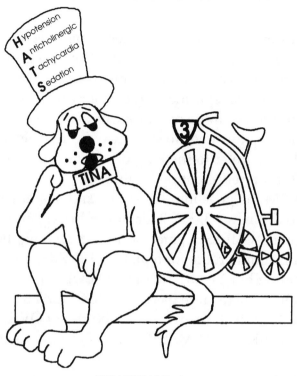

©2001 I CAN Publishing, Inc.

Trimipramine

I mipramine

Nortriptyline

Amitriptyline

MONOAMINE OXIDASE (MAO) INHIBITORS

A few examples of these antidepressant medications are Marplan, Nardil and Parnate. They are given to inhibit the enzyme, monoamine oxidase, which breaks down norepinephrine and serotonin, increasing the concentration of these neurotransmitters. To assist you in reviewing the foods to stay away from while on these medicines, refer to the king on the next page or think of a tyrant (representing tyramine).

At 4:30 P.M. he goes into his study, and sits down to an ice cold mug of BEER, 2 glasses of WINE, and a platter of aged CHEESE. Later on in the evening, he goes into his dining room for a plate of LIVERS, home made steaming hot YEAST ROLLS, a bowl of FIGS, a glass of COLA, and a large piece of CHOCOLATE pie. In the middle of the table, there are 7 bottles of OVER-THE-COUNTER COLD MEDICINES. Tyramine is in most of these.

If the client takes tyramine (or any of these foods or meds), while on the MAO, it will cause a HYPERTEN-SIVE CRISIS. This will be characterized by increased temperature, tremors, tachycardia and a marked elevation in the blood pressure.

Watch for strokes!

MONOAMINE OXIDASE (MAO) INHIBITORS

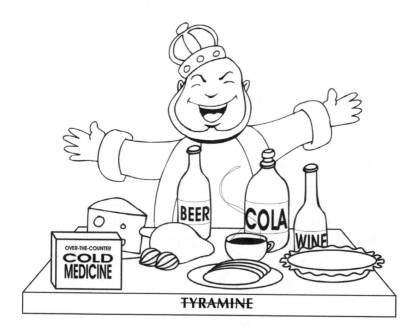

©1994 I CAN Publishing, Inc.

BIPOLAR DISORDER

This psychiatric challenge is very well named. Our clown is interestingly dressed on one side and quite shabbily dressed on the other. Unless these folks are treated, their behavior is at opposite ends of the pole. Sometimes they will be so UP that they are manic, and other times they are so DOWN in the dumps that they're ready to kill themselves.

When they are **UP**, they may think they are Elvis or some other magnificent person. They may think this 24 hours a day. They don't have time to rest, eat or sleep. Try giving them finger foods and providing noncompetitive activities to decrease their hyperactivity. Setting limits, being firm and helping them stay on Lithium may be the best approach. Lithium works best when there is a sodium balance, so try to find them something to do besides play football which is sure to make them sweat. (Besides, this is competitive–Talk about hyper!)

When they are **DOWN**, it's hard to please them. Everything is negative, nothing is right. They still do not eat or sleep well because they are too depressed. Suicide is a common problem. Maintain Lithium at 0.5-1.5 mEq/L. Report any assessment which will alter the sodium level. Other medications currently used to treat this process may include anticonvulsants, antipsychotics, and benzodiazepines.

GOOD LUCK!

BIPOLAR DISORDER

M ood elevated

A grandiose delusion

N eed for sleep, eat ↓

I nappropriate

C langing, loud, vulgar

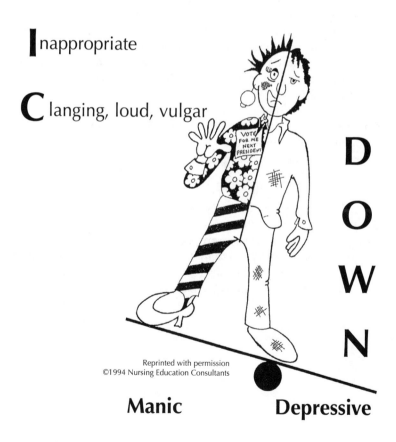

Reprinted with permission
©1994 Nursing Education Consultants

Manic　　　　　**Depressive**

LITHIUM

Lithium is used for the manic episode in biplolar disorder. It acts to lower concentrations of norepinephrine and serotonin by inhibiting their release. Maintenance lithium serum levels should be between .5–1.5 mEq/Liter. Blood tests need to initially be done weekly. Maintenance blood levels should be done one time per month. Lithium should be taken the same time each day preferably with meals or milk. Do not crush, chew, or break the extended-release or film coated tablets.

Laboratory studies of the **thyroid** hormone and periodic palpation of the thyroid gland should be a part of preventive therapy. Report signs of hypothyroidism. Symptoms are reversible when lithium is discontinued and supplemental thyroid is provided.

Polyuria or **incontinence**, mild **thirst**, fine **hand tremors** or jaw tremors may occur in early treatment of mania or sometimes persist throughout therapy. Usually however, symptoms subside with temporary reduction of dose. A neuromuscular reaction is **unsteady gait**.

Encourage a diet containing normal amounts of salt and a fluid intake of 3 liters per day. Assess clients who are high risk to develop toxicity such as postoperative, dehydration, hyperthyroidism, renal disease, or those clients taking diuretics.

You will find LITHIUM on Monitoring Lab Values by the Magic 2s.

Lithium was the first mood stabilizing drug approved by the U.S. Food and Drug Administration and is probably the most common drug used for bipolar disorder (see next page). Valproic acid (Depakote) and carbamazepine (Tegretol) are anti-convulsant drugs, yet also have a mood stabilizing effect. These drugs may be combined with Lithium or with each other for maximum effectiveness.

DRUG FOR MANIC CLIENT

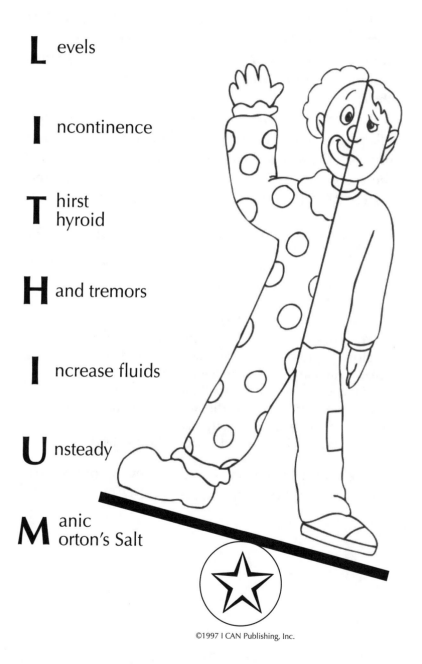

L evels

I ncontinence

T hirst
thyroid

H and tremors

I ncrease fluids

U nsteady

M anic
orton's Salt

SCHIZOPHRENIA

The schizophrenic disorders are **HARD** to deal with. Their behavior is often maladaptive and involves alterations in thinking, moods, feelings, perceptions, communication patterns and interpersonal relationships.

The schizophrenic client has a **HARD** time with relationships and a **HARD** time with the establishment of trust. The word "**HARD**" may help you remember these concepts. It's **HARD** being schizophrenic and it's **HARD** (challenging) providing nursing care.

The nurse said to the person with schizophrenia, "It's time for lunch."

He said, "I'm DEAD, Dead folks don't eat."

She said, "It's time for meds."

He said, "Dead folks don't take meds."

She said, "Time for a bath."

You guessed it. "Dead folks don't bathe either."

How to prove to him that he was not dead? She had a great idea! She asked, "Do dead folks bleed?"

"Of course dead folks don't bleed," he answered.

She went after her needle and syringe and took some blood from his arm, held it up proudly and said, "SEE!"

He said, "I'll be damned, dead folks do bleed."

The moral to this story is that they cannot be reasoned with and the nursing care is **HARD**.

SCHIZOPHRENIA

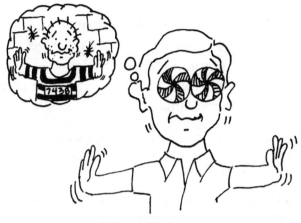

©1994 I CAN Publishing, Inc.

H allucinations

A ffect, ambivalence, autism,
associative looseness

R elationship

D elusions

UNDESIRABLE EFFECTS OF ANTIPSYCHOTIC DRUGS

People that take antipsychotic drugs may have a different **STANCE**. They may shuffle their feet or have other unusual symptoms while taking these mood-altering drugs. **STANCE** will help you remember many of these undesirable effects.

S **SEDATION**, sleepiness and **SUNLIGHT SENSITIVITY** are common with these drugs. Often they are not able to drive.

T **TARDIVE DYSKINESIA** is an irreversible effect that changes the stance because it changes the head.

A **ANTICHOLINERGIC** effects can make the client's mouth dry and can cause constipation. **AGRANULOCYTOSIS** is an undesirable effect. Report sore throats or signs of sepsis.

N **NEUROLEPTIC MALIGNANT SYNDROME** may occur.

C **CARDIAC EFFECTS** of orthostatic hypotension are common.

E **EXTRAPYRAMIDAL** effects such as pill rolling and akathesia may occur.

UNDESIRABLE EFFECTS OF ANTIPSYCHOTICS

S edation
unlight sensitivity

T ardive dyskinesia

A nticholinergic
granulocytosis

N euroleptic malignant syndrome

C ardiac arrhythmias (orthostatic hypotension)

E xtrapyramidal (akathesia)

ALCOHOLISM

One of the goals during the long-term rehabilitation is to assist client in identifying alternate coping mechanisms. "**COPES**" is the key in reviewing the priority nursing plans.

C **COPING MECHANISMS**–Encourage client to develop alternative coping mechanisms other than alcohol to deal with stress. The client must be responsible for sobriety.

O **ORIENT TO COMMUNITY RESOURCES**–Refer clients to available community resources such as Alcoholics Anonymous (AA), Alanon and Alateen. Abuse of spouses or children often occur while the client is drinking. Notify appropriate protection services for suspected spouse or child abuse.

P **PLAN** may include antabuse. Antabuse is a drug used by a willing client as a deterrent that will make the client violently ill (flushing, hypotension and nausea and vomiting if he takes it and drinks alcohol). The nurse should always know when the client had the last drink before she administers this drug. Never administer any medications or substances with alcohol in them (i.e., cough syrup, mouth wash, shaving cream, etc.) while the client is taking antabuse.

E **ENCOURAGE DIET**–Vitamin B complex is often used for the alcoholic client with delerium tremens and for the treatment of peripheral neuritis. Alcoholics often have avitaminosis because they drink instead of eat. Folic acid deficiency can lead to obstetrical complications.

S **SEIZURES**–Delerium Tremens usually occur within 48 hours after cessation of drinking. Picking at the bed covers, tremors of hands, anxiety, nausea, hypertension and nightmares followed by seizures may cause an emergency.

ALCOHOLISM

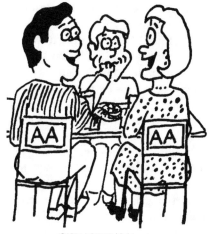

©1994 I CAN Publishing, Inc.

C oping mechanisms

O rient to community resources

P lan may include antabuse

E ncourage vitamin B, folic acid

S eizures

DEMENTIA

"The Slow House of Alzheimer's" tells the story of Poppa, who came to live with his son, but was so confused. The first night Son found Poppa a mile down the road in his pajama shirt and boxer shorts. He had fallen and his leg was bleeding. Poppa was "going to the house" (4 states away). To protect him, Son put a chair in front of his bedroom door, so that when he got up in the middle of the night he would be heard. Poppa would have gone nuts if he had been restrained. Barriers are much safer and more humane.

Son's wife could not wait to take Poppa to the cafeteria dining room so he could choose his own food, but Poppa stood there and stood there. Son's wife had to choose his food because decisions were impossible. The bathroom was a problem. Poppa had used the "out of doors" when he was a boy and his memory had regressed. It was easier to schedule his elimination than to embarrass the neighbors. Unfortunately the schedule was not always accurate and sometimes there were embarrassing wet clothes.

This story is a common one for people with dementia. **"The Slow House of Alzheimer's"** will help you remember the symptoms of lost and **wandering, confusion, decision difficulty, incontinence** and **confinement for safety**.

These changes are often progressive and irreversible. The cardinal rule for the geriatric population is do not push too fast (go slowly). It is important to reorient Poppa to the current **reality**. Objects such as clocks and calendars may help. Poppa's self-esteem may benefit through **reminiscing**. He may be able to recall events 10 years ago, but not 10 minutes ago. Poppa needs to be encouraged to remain **independent** as long as possible. Avoid dependency. Develop a plan for activities of daily living and remember consistency is important. As Poppa has illustrated, safety is very important. Due to sundowners and the increase risk of wandering and falling, **safety** precautions may become a high priority for these clients.

Remember–The difference between dementia (Alzheimer's) and delirium. Dementia is progressive and irreversible. Delirium or acute confusion state can result from sepsis, drug drug interactions, fluid and electrolyte imbalances, etc.

THE SLOW HOUSE OF ALZHEIMER'S

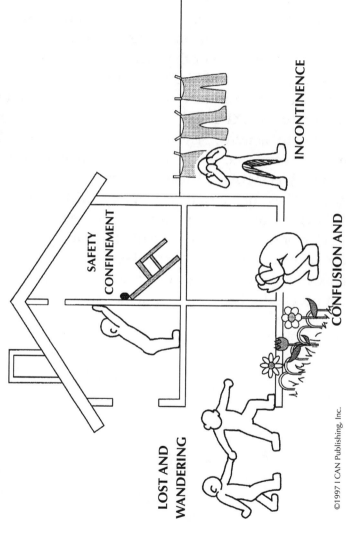

SAFETY CONFINEMENT

INCONTINENCE

CONFUSION AND DECISION DIFFICULTY

LOST AND WANDERING

©1997 I CAN Publishing, Inc.

LATER CHANGES IN DEMENTIA

Dementia is devastating to the client that knows something is "wrong," as well as heartbreaking to loved ones. The image on the next page will assist you in identifying some of the later changes in dementia. As you can see **APHASIA** is an issue with speech. They may not be able to talk or to understand. They may develop **APRAXIA** and lose their ability to perform purposeful activity. Sensory stimuli loss (**AGNOSIA**) may be common. The inability to remember certain items (**ANOMIA**) is frustrating and may make them angry. They may lose their memory (**AMNESIA**) and fail to recognize their spouse and children.

Dementia affects the client, the family and the caretakers. Remember, "caretakers die first". For this reason it is important that nurses help caretakers find support and relief from a demented loved one.

LATER CHANGES
WITH DEMENTIA

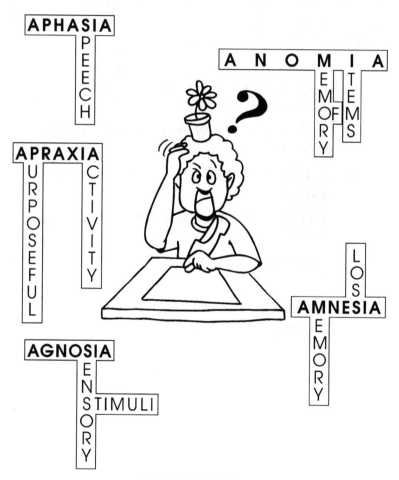

COMBATIVE CLIENT

Many people feel they put combat boots on the minute they get up in the morning, but we are referring to the client who is out of control. This may include folks that are real mad, manics, alcoholics, dementias and personality disorders just to name a few. It does not matter what the etiology is; the concept of "**COMBAT**" is still the same.

C   **CONTROL IMMEDIATE SITUATION**–Get their attention. Remove harmful objects. Maintain distance between self and client. Remain neutral.

O   **OUT OF SITUATION**–Remove client from the environment to de-escalate combative behavior.

M   **MAINTAIN CALM**–Do not hurry. Channel the agitated behavior.

B   **BE FIRM AND SET LIMITS**–Be consistent and prevent overt aggression.

A   **AVOID RESTRAINTS**–Use restraints as a last intervention.

T   **TRY CONSEQUENCES**–Positive consequences for positive behavior.

COMBATIVE CLIENT

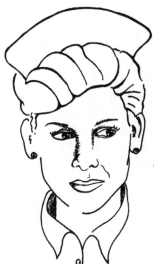

Control immediate

Out of situation

Maintain calm

Be firm/set limits

Avoid restraints

Try consequences

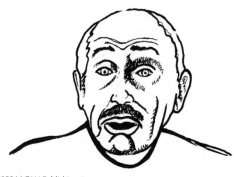

CULTURAL ASPECTS

Our world grows smaller as we visit and work in countries other than our own and as people from other cultures come to the United States to live and work. We are grateful to have had the opportunity to work with international nurses that have assisted us with using the word **SPIRIT** to bring together the commonalities in many of our cultures.

S **SOUL FOOD**–foods that are comfort foods for us are important to or forbidden by our culture or religion. Example–Many people of Italian descent love pasta, but when diagnosed with diabetes may have to severely limit pasta intake.

P **PRODUCTS** such as blood products, have different connotations to different cultures and religious groups. For example, the Jehovah's Witness Religion chooses to refuse blood and blood products. Alternative fluids and autologous transfusions may be acceptable

I **INTERACTIONS** in communication differ with many cultures. For example, South African people may love to entertain with song and dance while many Asians are shy and reserved. Native Americans may be offended with direct eye contact while American businessmen may be offended it there is no direct eye contact. Interpreters may need to be utilized to have effective communication when people are ill.

R **RITUALS** are a part of every culture, births, weddings, and funerals are time-honored events in most all cultures and may have any rituals associated with them. For example, some cultures choose to burn the umbilical cord when if falls off the infant to "keep the sins of the mother from being visited on the baby."

I **IN TRANSITION** from the body of life to the spiritual life is especially important for nurses. For example, Moslem men should be cared for after death only by another man.

T **TEACHING** health care promotion and prevention of illness may be challenging to many cultures that may value voodoo, Chinese herbs, medicine men and other kinds of treatment. Our nursing goal is to determine the cultural issues so that we can increase compliance with health care without offending global cultures while valuing their practices.

CULTURE

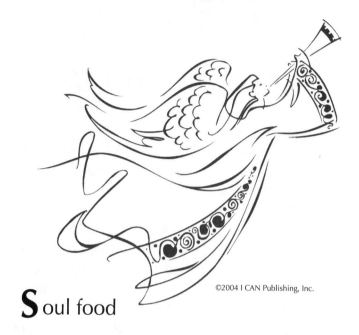

©2004 I CAN Publishing, Inc.

S oul food

P roducts (blood)

I nteractions (communication)

R ituals

I n transition

T eaching

SENSORY PERCEPTION

VISUAL CHANGES

The images on the next page will help you recall the major eye disorders. **GLAUCOMA** is described by clients as seeing halos around lights. Tunnel vision is another common complaint resulting from an increase in intraocular pressure. Loss of vision can occur. Glaucoma is chronic and a major cause of blindness.

CATARACT is a complete or partial opacity of the lens. This disorder is described as a decrease in visual acuity. Imagine you had on your sunglasses, and we took a paint brush and painted white paint on the outside of your glasses. Could you see out? Of course not. Is it painful? No. That is similar to cataracts.

RETINAL DETACHMENT is described as a sensation of having a veil or curtain over the eye. This disorder is sudden in onset. Some clients may experience an area of blank vision. Retinal detachment occurs from a separation of the two layers of the retina. When separation occurs, vitreous humor seeps between the layers and detachment of the retina from the choroid occurs.

MACULAR DEGENERATION is described as a blind spot in the center of the field of vision. Peripheral vision is retained but client is unable to read, drive, etc. There is no cure at this time.

VISUAL CHANGES

Glaucoma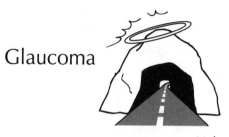

Halo tunnel

Cataracts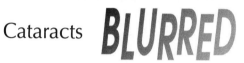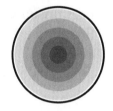

Blurred

Retinal detachment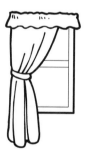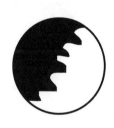

Curtain

Macular degeneration **BLACK SP⬤T**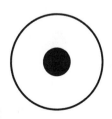

Black spot

SYMPTOMS OF OPEN ANGLE GLAUCOMA

The image on the next page shows a big cup (optic) in a tunnel (tunnel vision). The client with open angle glaucoma may occasionally see halos around lights. They experience a loss of peripheral vision, which creates this tunnel vision. The good news is that this is a painless condition. The bad news is that glaucoma is one of the leading causes of blindness. Although this condition is not an emergency, we want to help the clients prolong the effects of vision loss with medication. See the next page.

OPEN ANGLE GLAUCOMA

O ccasionally see halos around light

P eripheral vision (gradually lose)
ainless
rogressive vision loss

E arly stages asymptomatic
nlarged optic cup

N ot an emergency

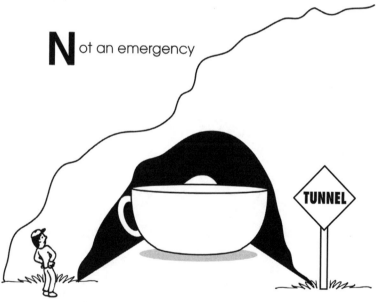

MEDICATIONS FOR OPEN ANGLE GLAUCOMA

Clients with glaucoma will experience an increase in intraocular pressure. They may feel as if there is a **"BAHM"** (a bomb going off in their eyes). Our bomb on the next page is pointed down because this is the direction that we want the intraocular pressure to go while our client is using these medications.

MEDICATIONS FOR OPEN ANGLE GLAUCOMA

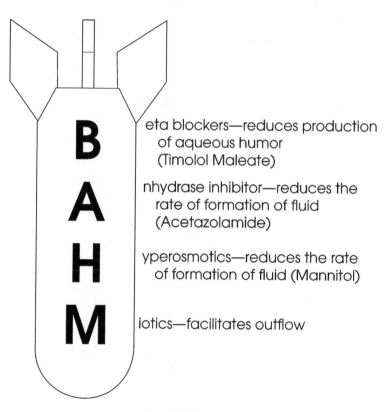

Beta blockers—reduces production of aqueous humor (Timolol Maleate)

Anhydrase inhibitor—reduces the rate of formation of fluid (Acetazolamide)

Hyperosmotics—reduces the rate of formation of fluid (Mannitol)

Miotics—facilitates outflow

MIOTICS

Miotics are given to people who have an elevated pressure in the eye due to glaucoma. The word miotics has a **C** in it for constrict. As a result of the constriction from these drugs, there is an increased flow of the aqueous humor. Interestingly enough, many of the miotic eye drops contain the word **CAR**. **CARpine**, **CARbachol**, and **piloCARpine** are all miotics.

Notice the tag on our friend's car. He "*KANT C*" well due to his tunnel vision. Clients with primary open-angle glaucoma experience a gradual loss of peripheral vision which is described as "tunnel vision."

Isn't that EASY?

CONSTRICT EYES: GLAUCOMA

MIOTICS

C
O
N O ATROPINE!!
S
T
R
I
C
T

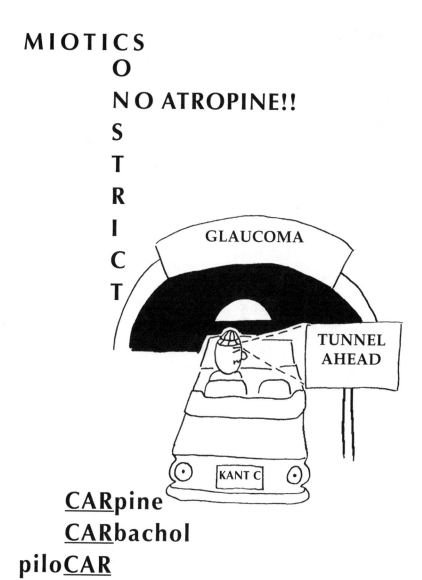

CARpine
CARbachol
pilo**CAR**

EAR DROPS

Aren't these guys great! They epitomize Accelerated Learning.

The ear canal changes as we grow. To be sure that ear drops can get down into the ear, we need to remember how to hold the ear when we're putting in those drops. Notice the word *adult* has a **U** in it for **UP**. Hold the adult ear **UP** and back. Notice that the word *child* ends in a **D**. Hold the child's ear **DOWN** and back.

WHEN INSTALLING EAR DROPS
REMEMBER THAT THE EAR IS

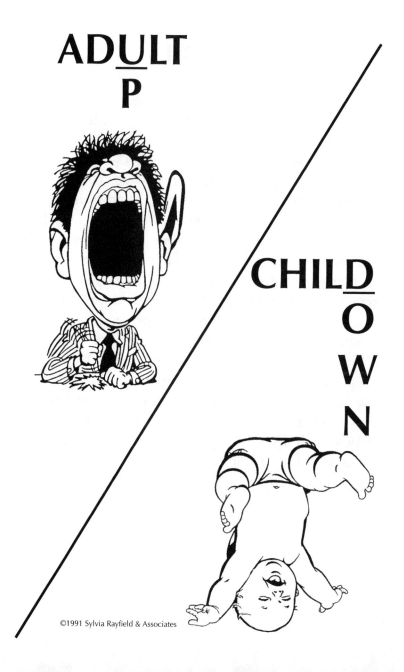

ADU̲LT
P

CHIL̲D
O
W
N

ENDOCRINE

SIADH

Soggy Sid has SIADH (syndrome of inappropriate antidiuretic hormone), a condition that continually releases the antidiuretic hormone (ADH). With increased ADH, the body retains water and gets so Soggy that water intoxication may occur.

Sid's cap is hiding his bandaged head from a head injury, which is a major risk factor for SIADH. Due to his cerebral edema, he is prone to seizures. Notice his limbs are small. There is no obvious edema, yet he has gained weight in his body. The intake and output record will document low urinary output because he's keeping it all on board. The urine specific gravity will be high. The serum sodium will be decreased (dilutional). Limit Soggy Sid's fluid intake. He may be given diuretics to assist with fluid excretion, especially if he has respiratory or cardiac problems. Keep Soggy Sid's bed flat or only slightly elevated. This position of his head will decrease the secretion of ADH. Keep the neuro checks going. Soggy Sid is in serious condition!

SOGGY SID

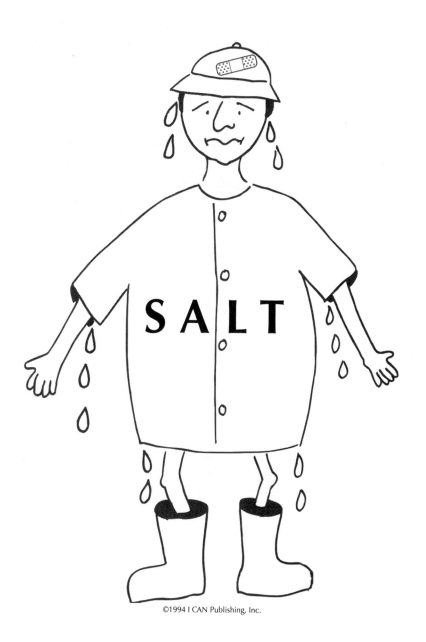

DIABETES INSIPIDUS

Due to a lack of pitressin excretion from the Pituitary gland, our poor dried-up California prune is shriveled up because he urinates a lot (polyuria). This loss of body fluids will cause him to be very dehydrated and have a low specific gravity in his urine. To monitor Mr. Prune, the nurse will need to keep accurate daily weights and watch his vital signs.

Offer him plenty to drink and keep a watch on his specific gravity. He may require IV fluids for rehydration. This guy can get dehydrated in a hurry and must be watched closely.

DIABETES INSIPIDUS

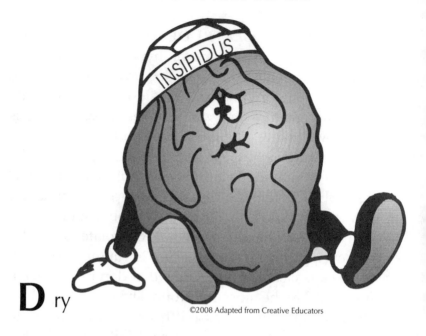

D ry

©2008 Adapted from Creative Educators

I + O, daily weight

L ow specific gravity

U rinates lots

T reat = pituitary hormone

r **E** hydrate

HYPERTHYROIDISM

GO GETTER GERTRUDE will help you remember the major symptoms of hyperthyroidism. Her last name, of course, is Graves. Graves' disease is the result of hyperthyroidism. One look at this visually stunning creature, and you can see how thin she is and how her eyes "bug out" (exophthalmus). Everything is running except her menstrual periods. Her HEART is running fast (increased pulse), her BLOOD PRESSURE is running UP, and her basal metabolic rate (BMR) is running, therefore the metabolism of drugs will be faster. She can eat a whole chocolate cake without ever gaining an ounce. She is running so much that she is cleaning out closets that don't need cleaning at 3:00 in the morning. Notice she is wearing short sleeves and pants because it takes a lot of energy to run, and she is hot all the time. While planning her nursing care, lower the room temperature and get rid of all those excess blankets. A quiet room will be great! Well-balanced meals (high in calories and vitamins) is a must. Due to the eye changes, protect cornea from drying. GO GETTER'S diagnostic tests would reveal an increase in the following reports: T3 and T4, protein bound iodine (PBI), BMR, and uptake of I 131. (Refer to **Hypothyroidism.**)

GO GETTER GERTRUDE

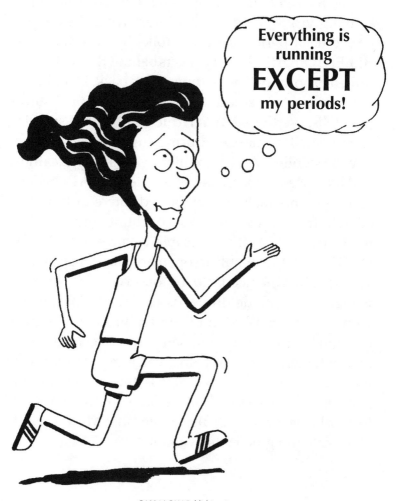

THYROIDECTOMY

The **BOW TIE** is around his neck because the hyperactive thyroid gland has been removed. Post-op can be a crucial period for these folks because they may **BLEED**. Often the blood collects behind the neck, being pulled by gravity if he is lying on his back. Place him in semi-Fowler's position to avoid tension on the suture line. Observe the **AIRWAY** due to potential swelling from being traumatized during surgery. Vocal chords may be swollen. Assess frequently for noisy breathing and increased restlessness. Evaluate **VOCAL** changes; increasing hoarseness may be indicative of laryngeal edema. If these people get into trouble they can lose their airway fast. It's advisable to have a **TRACHE-OTOMY SET** available to open an emergency airway. The **INCISION** needs to be observed for swelling which can occlude the airway. Watch for normal wound healing. We don't want an infection. Evaluate calcium levels; parathyroids may have been damaged or accidentally removed. Since calcium potentiates the movement of electrolytes across the cell membrane and electrolyte balance is imperative for the heart cells to work, low levels could create an **EMERGENCY**. Have calcium gluconate available!

POST-OP THYROIDECTOMY

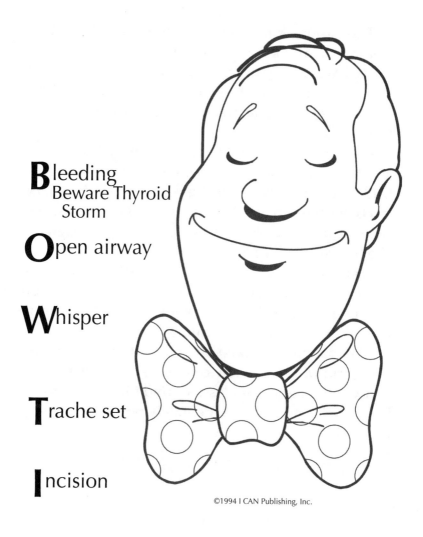

Bleeding
   Beware Thyroid
   Storm

Open airway

Whisper

Trache set

Incision

Emergency

©1994 I CAN Publishing, Inc.

HYPOTHYROIDISM

This vision of loveliness is **MORBID MATILDA**. Her last name, as you've probably guessed, is Myxedema (Hypothyroid). She has a slow deterioration of the thyroid function. It occurs mostly in older adults and five times more frequently in women than in men.

As you can see, Matilda has the family "bug-eyes" and she has no menstrual period like her sister Gertrude, but that's where the resemblance ends. (Refer to **Hyperthyroidism**.) Matilda is not thin. In fact, she can look at a piece of chocolate cake and gain weight. She had rather sleep at 3:00 in the morning than clean closets. She may also be sleeping at 3:00 in the afternoon because of her lack of energy. Her long pants and putting her hands in her pocket will keep her warm. Increasing the room temperature may be necessary.

Matilda will be placed on lifelong thyroid replacement, and will be on a low-calorie, low cholesterol diet to help with her weight loss. Morbid Matilda does not like these changes. She is definitely not a very happy camper!

MORBID MATILDA

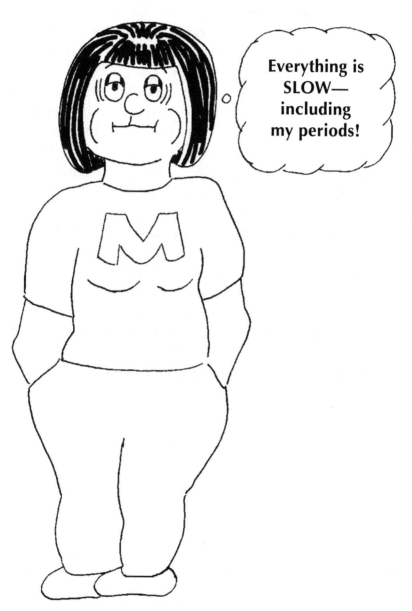

DIABETES MELLITUS

FIDO, the diabetic dog, is exhibiting all of the signs and symptoms of hyperglycemia. Sugar is floating around in his blood stream because there is no insulin to take the sugar into the cells.

Since the cells are starving for lack of sugar, Fido is dreaming of food. He has a huge appetite. His food bowl in front of him remains empty because he keeps trying to feed those starving cells (POLYPHAGIA). The high sugar content in his blood is pulling fluid from the cells which makes him very thirsty (POLYDIPSIA). Since his kidneys are compensating by dumping extra fluid and sugar out onto the street (POLYURIA), he has totally wet down the fire hydrant. Look at Fido's pants! They don't fit any more. The sugar and the fluid that he has taken in have not gone into his cells, since there is no insulin to assist in crossing over into the cell. As a result, poor Fido has LOST WEIGHT. What medication would you plan to have available? Insulin of course. (Refer to **Hypoglycemia**.)

WHAT'S WRONG WITH FIDO?

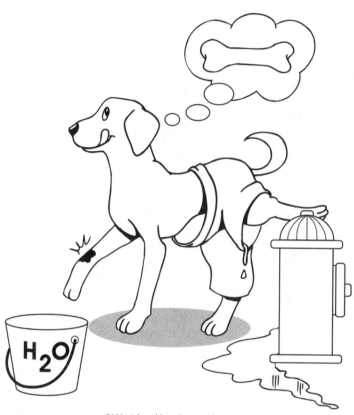

©1994 Adapted from Creative Educators

INSULIN

Do you have difficulty remembering the onset, peak, and duration of the various types of insulin? Let us help simplify this for you, so it will be easy!! In your mind it will be helpful to categorize the rapid, intermediate, and long acting insulin. The onset of the regular insulin is 30–60 minutes. The onset of humalog is < 15 minutes. If you can recall this time frame being real fast, then you will be able to remember the other insulins. For the intermediate insulin, multiply 60 x 2 and the onset is 60–120 minutes. For the long acting insulin, multiply 120 x 2 and the onset is 240 min.–320 min.

As you can see on caps on the next page, the peak has a general progression. Regular starts with a peak of 3 hours. Multiply 3 x 2 to get a peak of 6–12 hours for the intermediate insulin. As you can see the long acting insulin's peak is increased to 8–20 hrs. (remember 6 + 2 = 8). These will assist you in remembering the average peak action for your examination.

The duration of Humalog is 4 hrs. The remainder of the times are in increments of 6. The regular insulin's duration is 6 hrs. Multiply that by 3 and the intermediate insulin is 18–24 hrs. The long acting insulin has the longest duration of 36 hrs. See **HYPOGLYCEMIA** for insulin reaction.

Lantus is a long acting insulin. It has an onset of 1.1 hrs. There is no peak and it has a duration of 24 hrs.

Remember–Regular insulin is the only insulin which may be given IV.

PEAK TIMES FOR INSULIN

LONG
ONSET
240–320 MINUTES

INTERMEDIATE
ONSET 60–120
MINUTES

COMBINATION
ONSET 30–60 MINUTES
THEN 1–2 HOURS

SHORT
ONSET 30–60 MINUTES
(HUMALOG: <15 MIN)

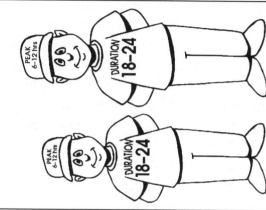

PEAK
8–20 hrs

DURATION
36

ULTRA HUMULIN

PEAK
6–12 hrs

DURATION
18–24

LENTE

PEAK
6–12 hrs

DURATION
18–24

NPH

PEAK
6–12 hrs

DURATION
18–24

PEAK
2–4 hrs

DURATION
6–8

REGULAR/NPH

PEAK
3 hrs

DURATION
6–8

REGULAR

PEAK
1 hr

DURATION
4

HUMALOG

©2001 I CAN Publishing, Inc.

HYPOGLYCEMIA

People taking insulin may have hypoglycemic reactions. This is a fact. Some diabetics have them everyday; others rarely have this problem. Teach them the symptoms, so they recognize their situation. Some of the signs and symptoms to observe are they may get suddenly **TIRED** and run out of steam. **TACHYCARDIA** (rapid pulse) occurs as a warning. **TREMORS** or nervousness are other warning signs. They often become **IRRITABLE** and **RESTLESS**. They may mow anyone down in the coke line to get some food due to **EXCESSIVE HUNGER**. They know if they don't, they may be out! **DIAPHORESIS** is common, and is an excellent guideline for determining if the client is asleep versus having a hypoglycemic reaction. If the client is unconscious, administer glucagon IV. Encourage them to eat carbohydrates or drink milk if they are awake.

*If ever in doubt of a diagnosis of hypoglycemia versus hyperglycemia, give carbohydrates–severe hypoglycemia can result in permanent brain damage.

Remember this jingle to help recall the differences:

COLD AND CLAMMY MEANS YOU NEED SOME CANDY HOT AND DRY MEANS YOUR SUGAR IS HIGH.

Jingle reprinted with permission, NEC, Dallas, Texas

SYMPTOMS OF HYPOGLYCEMIA

Tremors
achycardia

Irritability

Restless

Excessive hunger

Diaphoresis
epression

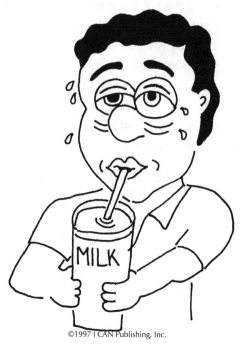

CUSHING'S SYNDROME

One look at **CUSHY CARL** and you see his problem. He has an overproduction of hormones from the adrenal cortex. As you see, he's holding a "twinkie." These people may have a HIGH BLOOD SUGAR. The bag of chips he is holding indicates his INCREASE in SODIUM resulting in fluid retention. Increase in volume naturally will ELEVATE the BLOOD PRESSURE. Watch that POTASSIUM level, it will have a tendency to DECREASE and we certainly do not want his heart doing any strange dances (arrhythmias). Cushy's fat face also let's us know he's holding fluids. His "buffalo hump" probably scares him enough that his blood pressure goes up even higher. The sore on his leg won't heal because of his high blood sugar. (Would we want to protect him from INFECTION? You bet!)

Put 2 and 2 together. Would we want to give a diabetic steroids? Not if we can help it. Sometimes there are no options, so if this is the case, monitor the blood sugar. Now we know that cortisone (steroids) will increase the blood sugar even higher, increase edema, and increase the risk for infection. With all of this going on, Cushy will indeed need some assistance with his emotional state.

We know we would! What about you?

CUSHY CARL

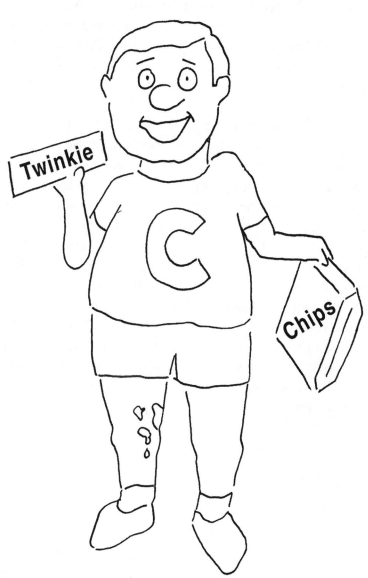

ADDISON'S DISEASE

ANEMIC ADAM, whose last name is Addison, is Cushy Carl's half brother. (Refer to **Cushing's Syndrome**.) The whole family thinks they have opposite characteristics. Adam has a disorder which is caused by a decrease in secretion of the adrenal cortex hormone.

Adam craves salt since he doesn't have enough. That is the reason he is out in the field at the salt lick. Hyponatremia has a tendency to cause low blood pressure. In addition, his potassium may be increased. He has hypoglycemia and complains of being tired and weak much of the time. This weakness is a cardinal complaint and usually is more severe in times of stress. Occasionally, Adam stays in bed. After his anorexia, nausea, vomiting and diarrhea, he is dehydrated and has a serious loss in weight. After all of this, who wouldn't be tired and weak? His skin has turned bronze, and it is not due to too much sun. This is caused by increased levels of melanocyte stimulating hormone (MSH). To prevent addisonian crisis, corticosteroids will have to be replaced.

ANEMIC ADAM

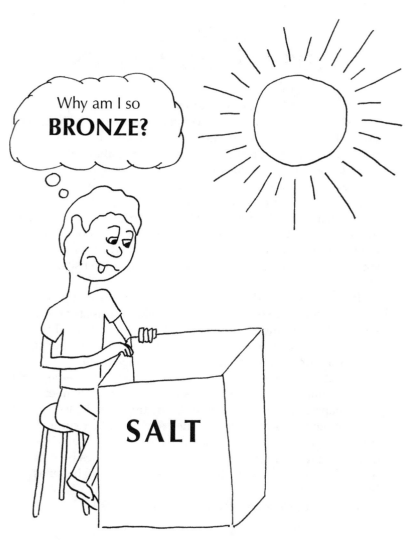

CARDIAC SYSTEM

TOOLS OF PHYSICAL ASSESSMENT

The tools of Physical Assessment are the most important in assessing, evaluating and monitoring the client's care. The appropriate tools include inspection, auscultation, percussion and palpation. Inspection is the use of the eyes to gather data. Careful observation can reveal clues about the client's respiratory system, musculoskeletal and neurological system, skin integrity, and the emotional and mental status.

Auscultation is the process of listening to sounds produced by the organs and tissues of the body. It is a clinical tool used most frequently to assess the heart, lungs, neck and abdomen. These sounds are characterized according to pitch, intensity, quality and duration.

Percussion is used for assessing the size, position and density of underlying structures. This technique consists of a sharp tapping that produces vibrations and subsequent sound waves. These sound waves are interpreted by the experienced percussor as air, fluid or solid material in an underlying structure.

Palpation is the use of hands and fingers to gather data through touch. The characteristics of body texture, temperature, size, shape and movement may be distinguished by different parts of the hands and fingers. The palm and ulnar surfaces are used to distinguish vibrations and the dorsal surface is best for estimating temperature. A bimanual technique uses both hands to entrap an organ or mass between the fingertips to better assess its size and shape.

Practice, practice and practice improve this skill.

TOOLS OF
PHYSICAL ASSESSMENT

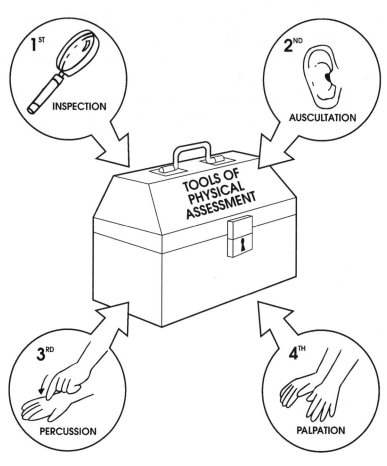

STETHOSCOPE

The stethoscope is indispensable for determining the sounds inside the body. The image on the next page will assist you in determining when to use the diaphragm or the bell of the stethoscope to hear the best sounds.

The diaphragm is used to hear high pitched heart sounds such as S_1 and S_2, murmurs of aortic and mitral valve regurgitation, pericardial, and abdominal friction rub sounds.

The bell is used to hear lower pitched heart sounds such as S_3, S_4 and a murmur of mitral stenosis.

THE STETHOSCOPE

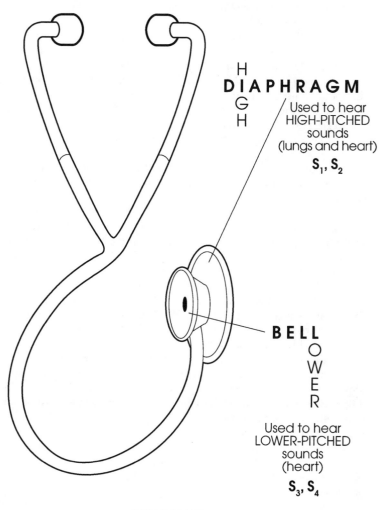

H
G
H
DIAPHRAGM
Used to hear
HIGH-PITCHED
sounds
(lungs and heart)
S_1, S_2

BELL
O
W
E
R

Used to hear
LOWER-PITCHED
sounds
(heart)
S_3, S_4

VITAL SIGNS

Vital signs are just that. **VITAL to LIFE**. If we have no BP, inspiration, temperature or pulse, we are dead. That makes these the most important assessments that a nurse can make. A flow sheet on a history of vital signs will give the nurse valuable information on which to make life-saving decisions.

The ordinary definition of a normal blood pressure varies with the client, but can range around 120/80. If the client has hypertension, the nurse may hear the BP over 200/100. This high a BP is a priority for the nurse to take action as it is "stroke territory." Clients on BP medication must be taught to monitor their own BP to make sure it stays within a normal range (usually below 140/80).

Cuff size is important in determining an accurate BP. For example, do not use a neonatal cuff (2" wide) on a 250-pound man. It may cut his arm, and the reading will be inaccurate. "Hard cuffs" commonly found on automatic BP readers, often leave big bruises on little old ladies that are taking coumadin. Be cautious when taking the BP of the client on blood thinners.

LOC (level of consciousness) is essential as all vital signs may be within normal limits, but the client may be unresponsive and unconscious.

Breathing is a must. *"Assessment of the breath includes the number of times that we breathe per minute = respiratory rate).* An adult's respiratory rate is approximately 20 times per minute. *(Refer to the chart on the next page for respiratory rate change at different ages.)* If an adult has a high respiratory rate, they may not be exchanging air. High or low rate (under 12) is a high priority for nursing action. We also want to determine if the client is having difficulty breathing by assessing for dyspnea or shortness of breath (SOB). Is there a scared look on their face? Are they using chest and neck muscles to breathe? Does it hurt for them to breathe? These are vital assessments!

Skin assessment provides us with a lot of information. We can determine if they are hot, dry, cold or clammy. Assessing the body temperature is confirmation of what we feel. We can also determine if they are shivering by touching them. Maybe one of the most important things that we are doing is touching them to let them know that we care and to calm them.

Evaluating the pulse involves the heart rate *(around 70-80 for an adult, check chart for changes in other age groups).* While we are feeling the pulse, we can tell if it is regular, irregular, bounding, thready, strong or weak. An abnormal pulse is a high priority for nursing action.

Evaluating for pain is also a priority because it may result in vital sign changes. When people are hurting, their pulse and respiratory rate elevates. In fact, the pulse is a good indication for evaluating the effectiveness of pain medication.

VITAL SIGNS

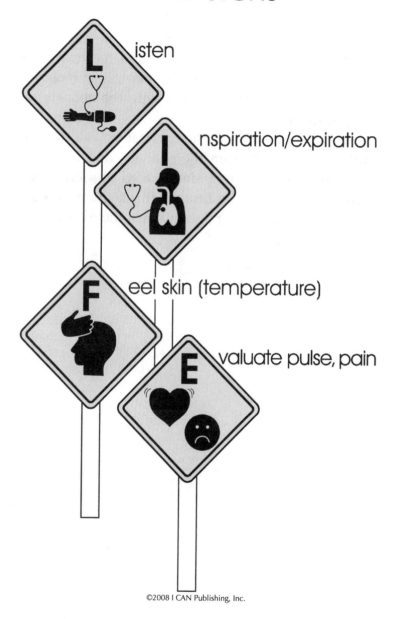

Listen

Inspiration/expiration

Feel skin (temperature)

Evaluate pulse, pain

*The vital signs on this page will assist you in remembering
what assessments are vital to "LIFE"!*

VITAL SIGN VALUES

Many learners indicate they have a hard time remembering the respiratory rate and the heart rate for the various stages of development. It in reality is quite simple! All you do is start with the neonate for your guidelines.

In order to determine the respiratory rate for the toddler, subtract 10 from the neonate, and the heart rate for the toddler can be determined by subtracting 20 from the neonate. Continue in this fashion for each of the stages. The next page outlines the averages to validate your figures.

Now, was that so hard?

VITAL SIGN VALUES

Neonate

Respiratory	40
Heart Rate	140

Toddler (age 2–4)

Respiratory	30
Heart Rate	120

Child (6–10)

Respiratory	20
Heart Rate	100

Adult

Respiratory	12–18
Heart Rate	60–100

CARDIAC SOUNDS

Cardiac sounds are one effective assessment for identifying alterations in the cardiaovascular system. S_1 is ordinarily auscultated over the tricuspid/mitral sites. It is heard in the beginning of the cardiac cycle (systole) and is described as the sound "Lubb".

S_2 is auscultated over the pulmonic/aortic site. It is heard at the end of the cardiac cycle (diastole). This sound is described as "Dubb".

S_3 is usually ascultated over the apex in the left side-lying position. It is heard in early diastole. The sound is described as "Ken-tuck-y." Hearing the S_3 may indicate heart failure, which also has 3 syllables (heart fail-ure).

S_4 can be auscultated over the apex in the left side-lying position. It is heard in late diastole and is described as "Tenn-e-see." Hearing the S_4 may indicate hypertension, which also has 4 syllables (hy-per-ten-sion). The PMI or Point of Maximal Intensity is usually ascultated midline at the 5th intercostal space.

CARDIAC SOUNDS

NORMAL

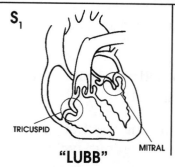

S₁

TRICUSPID

MITRAL

"LUBB"
Closure of
mitral and tricuspid valves

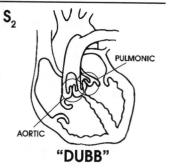

S₂

PULMONIC

AORTIC

"DUBB"
Closure of
aortic and pulmonic valves

ABNORMAL

S₃

**Heart Fail-ure
(3 syllables)**
Physiologic
(usually in children and young
adults)

S₄

**Hy-per-ten-sion
(4 syllables)**

DIAGNOSTICS
CARDIAC SYSTEM

Diagnostic testing MEETS a very big requirement in making cardiac diagnosis possible. A safe nurse will be able to answer these 3 questions about each of these Diagnostic Tests.

1. What should be completed prior to this test? (consent, teaching, allergies, holding meds, or food)

2. What should happen during this test? (positioning, anesthesia, invasive/noninvasive)

3. What should happen after this test? (reporting, monitoring)

DIAGNOSTICS
CARDIAC SYSTEM

M MRI (Determine claustrophobia and metal)

E EKG (Initiate, maintain, monitor, and intervene)

E Echocardiogram (Noninvasive)

T Thallium Uptake (NPO except H_2O/ no caffeine)

S Stress Test noninvasive

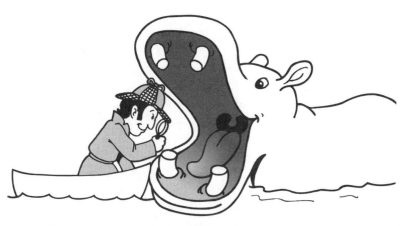

CYANOTIC HEART DEFECTS

Some folks have a hard time remembering which of those congenital heart defects are cyanotic versus which are acyanotic.

NO PROBLEM, just remember all congenital heart defects that begin with the letter "T" are cyanotic defects. Color the "T" on the next page blue to help you remember this easy concept.

FOUR T'S

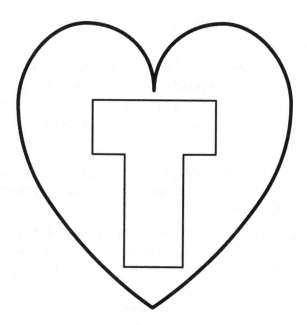

T etralogy

T runcus

T ransposition

T ricuspid

TETRALOGY OF FALLOT

Tetralogy of Fallot is often referred to as that complicated congenital heart defect that causes children to "squat" or "**DROP**" to the floor. When they get tired or out of breath, this position will decrease the amount of venous return to the heart. **DROP** will assist you in reviewing the four physiological defects with the heart in Tetralogy of Fallot.

D **DISPLACED AORTA** which allows unoxygenated blood into the oxygenated system causing cyanosis (overriding aorta).

R **RIGHT VENTRICLE HYPERTROPHIES** due to working so hard pumping against pressure. The more the heart muscle works the bigger it gets.

O **OPENING IN THE SEPTUM** is a "hole" that allows shunting of unoxygenated blood to mix with oxygenated blood (ventricular septal defect).

P **PULMONARY VALVE** partially closes making the right ventricle work, thus causing the right ventricle to hypertrophy.

These children are often small, tired, delicate and need surgery before leading a better quality of life. Teach parents to pace the child's activities, provide good nutrition to build strength and to renew themselves. Due to the challenges of these children, the parents need emotional support!

TETRALOGY OF FALLOT

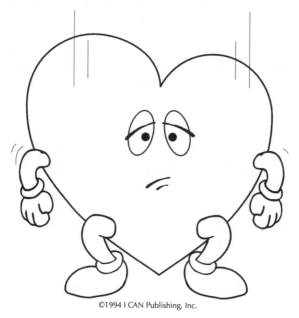

©1994 I CAN Publishing, Inc.

Displaced aorta

Right ventricle hypertrophy

Opening in septum

Pulmonary valve stenosis

ASSESSMENTS FOR CONGENITAL HEART DISEASE

This is to assist with remembering the nursing evaluation for an infant who has a serious defect requiring home care prior to corrective surgery. Think of a **HEART** since this is the location of surgery.

H **HEART MURMUR**–A murmur will be assessed especially with ventricular septal defects (VSD), atrial septal defects (ASD), and patent ductus arteriosus (PDA).

E **EVALUATE WEIGHT GAIN**–Due to their intolerance to suck well, they will have a slow weight gain. Some of these infants will be fed via a feeding tube because of their weakness.

A **ACTIVITY INTOLERANCE**–The infant fatigues easily. Conserve oxygen by anticipating their needs, so they won't cry.

R **RESPIRATORY INFECTIONS**–Due to pooling of blood in the pulmonary region, these infants have an increased frequency in respiratory infections.

T **TACHYCARDIA**–An elevation in the resting heart and respiratory rate are signs of hypoxia. Assess these changes carefully! They will give you a lot of information.

S **SUPPORT**–Allow family to grieve over loss of perfect infant. Foster early parent-infant attachment; encourage touching, holding and loving.

HEARTS

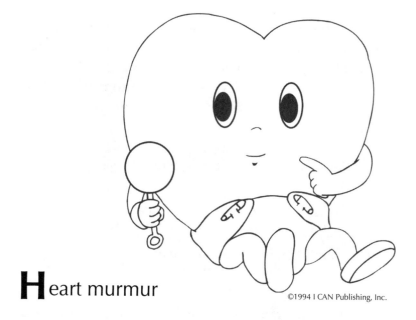

©1994 I CAN Publishing, Inc.

H eart murmur

E valuate weight

A ctivity intolerance

R espiratory infections

T achycardia & Tachypnea

S upport

HYPERTENSION

Catapres, a commonly used antihypertensive, is the name of our image to review RISK FACTORS. Just look at this gorgeous black woman. (Studies show that women of color have hypertension more often than other races.) See letters on the next page as you read below.

C People with hypertension may have small capillary hemorrhages in their eyes, blurred vision, and headaches.

A Nose bleeds could occur causing anxiety which leads to a further blood pressure increase.

T Carotid endarterectomies may be performed to prevent or relieve symptoms of a CVA caused from atherosclerosis of arteries in the throat.

A Her wide girth, obesity and hypertension go hand in hand. Remember, skinny, white chicks have high BP, too.

P Pheochromocytoma and adrenal tumors can cause hypertension.

R Notice the feet; diabetics are known to have hypertension. Thickened toe nails and foot ulcers may result in gangrene.

E E stands for "Essential" hypertension (unknown cause). Early high blood pressure may have few symptoms.

S Sexual dysfunction may occur as a result from the medicines.

HEALTH PROMOTION IS A MUST!

CATAPRES

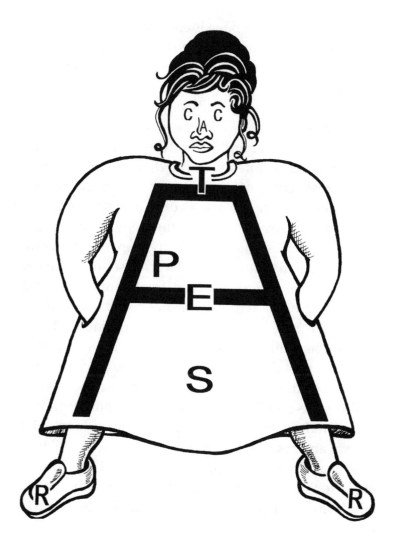

REDUCE CARDIAC WORKLOAD

The car on the next page is carrying a **SPARE** "heart tire." The goal for nursing care is to decrease the stress and strain on the heart after a myocardial infarction. *(It is the same as our goal when we drive our automobile; we do not want our tire to be damaged. The spare tire never quite replaces the original.)* After a myocardial infarction, modification in diet and lifestyle are important nursing implications. Lifestyle and diet changes should include **restriction of sodium and saturated fat** and a reduction or avoidance of alcohol consumption. It is important to **provide a calm**, quiet environment and comfort measures to ensure effectiveness of pain medications. Immediately after a MI the nurse should allow the client time to rest between treatments, and limit visitors and extra activity. Cardiac **after load** can be decreased by medications such as vasodilators. These medications will relax the vascular smooth muscle, producing vasodilation of the arterioles which reduces the cardiac after load. Anxiety can increase the oxygen requirements significantly; therefore, it is important to **reduce anxiety** in the client's life and encourage **daily renewal and rest**. This is an important time in a client's life to learn new relaxation techniques. The ultimate goal is for the client to return to his/her activities of daily living and to live a happy, healthy, productive life!

REDUCE CARDIAC WORKLOAD

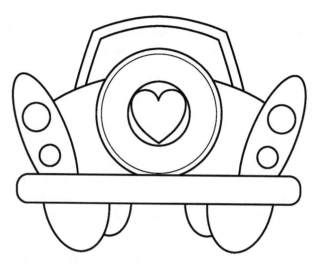

©1997 I CAN Publishing, Inc.

Sodium and saturated fat intake

Provide a calm environment

After load reduced

Reduce anxiety

Emotional rest

CARDIAC MANAGEMENT

OANM will assist you in remembering medications to administer to clients with chest pain.

O **OXYGEN** Oxygen will reduce complications from ischemia.

A **ASPIRIN** Aspirin is administered for its blood-thinning properties.

N **NITROGLYCERINE** Nitroglycerine will increase the blood supply to the heart by dilating the coronary arteries. The cardiac workload is reduced due to decrease in venous return as a result of the peripheral vasodilation.

M **MORPHINE** This analgesic will reduce the pain, which subsequently will decrease the ischemia.

Remember: If you need to prioritize, OANM will do it. Oxygen first, Aspirin second, Nitro, and then Morphine.

CARDIAC MANAGEMENT

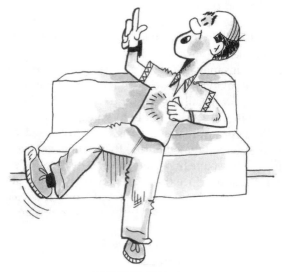

©2011 I CAN Publishing, Inc.

Oxygen

Aspirin

Nitroglycerine

Morphine

ACE INHIBITORS

What is an ACE Inhibitor?

It lowers blood pressure by stopping the angiotensin converting enzyme (ACE) in the lung, which reduces the vasoconstrictor, angiotensin II. This indeed will lower your blood pressure.

How do I remember all of these medications?

It's actually insanely easy!!! Let us introduce you to the "**Pril**" sisters who are taking a "**strol**" through the park to prevent cardiac problems. Strol will assist you to remember the actions of the ACE inhibitors. "**CHF**" will help you in remembering some undesirable effects from these drugs. CHF is used as a mnemonic to assist you in remembering that a client can receive these medications if they have hypertension and have experienced congestive heart failure. Since these drugs work directly at blocking the angiotensin converting enzyme (ACE), and it does not work directly on the heart, then these drugs are appropriate for clients with CHF.

What are some examples of these drugs?

> Capto**pril**
> Enala**pril**
> Lisino**pril**
> Fosino**pril**
> Rami**pril**
> Benzae**pril**

What do I need to evaluate?

1. Blood pressure - Since these medications reduce vasoconstriction, the pressure may go down too low. Observe for dizziness and/or tachycardia.

2. Some undesirable effects include an annoying dry cough, angioedema of the face, lips, tongue, and pharynx. Uncommon side effects include rash and taste distur- bances.

3. Monitor for hyponatremia and hyperkalemia.

4. With Captopril, agranulocytosis or neutropenia may occur (ask about sore throats).

PRIL SISTERS

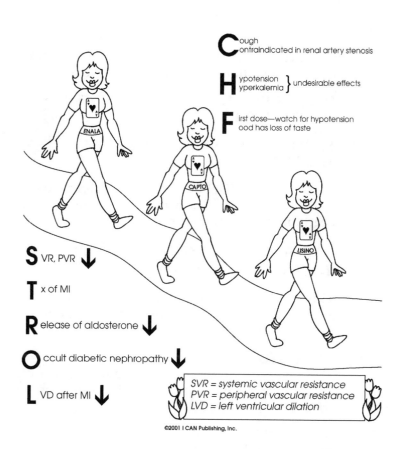

C ough
ontraindicated in renal artery stenosis

H ypotension
yperkalemia } undesirable effects

F irst dose—watch for hypotension
ood has loss of taste

S VR, PVR ↓

T x of MI

R elease of aldosterone ↓

O ccult diabetic nephropathy ↓

L VD after MI ↓

SVR = systemic vascular resistance
PVR = peripheral vascular resistance
LVD = left ventricular dilation

BETA BLOCKERS

Beta Blockers are a group of drugs that can be remembered using the acronym BETA. People taking these drugs may need TLC (tender loving care) because they may become drowsy or fatigued.

B **BROCHOSPASM** (so we don't want to give them to people with asthma or brochoconstrictive disease!)

E **ELICITS A DECREASE IN CARDIAC OUTPUT AND CONTRACTILITY.**

T **TREATS HYPERTENSION /ANGINA/ MIGRAINES/PANIC ATTACKS.**

A **AV CONDUCTION DECREASES** (short for treats arrhythmias, especially fast ones by decreasing the heart rate and cardiac output!)

**REMEMBER–STOP BETA BLOCKERS
WITH BRONCHOCONSTRICTIVE DISEASE**

T **TENORMIN** (atenolol) used for hypertension and angina (watch for renal impairment as this drug is renally excreted).

L **LOPRESSOR** (metoptolol) used for hypertension and angina (contraindicated in sinus bradycardia, 2nd or 3rd degree block, metabolized in liver and NOT renally excreted).

C **CORGARD** (nadolol) used for hypertension and angina (renally excreted, contraindicated in bronchial asthma, sinus bradycardia or 2nd or 3rd degree heart block).

NOTICE ALL THE GENERIC NAMES END IN "LOL"!

ROAD BLOCKS
TO BETA BLOCKERS

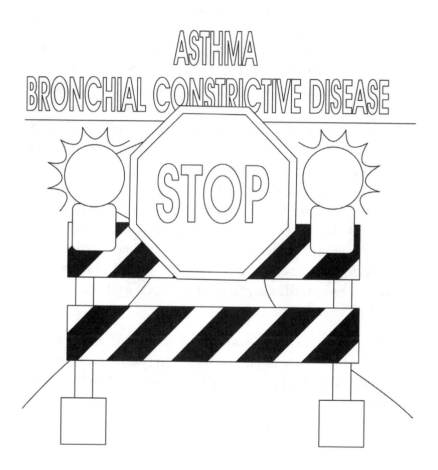

CALCIUM CHANNEL BLOCKERS

Calcium Channel Blockers are used to treat hypertension, angina, and migraine headaches. This group of medications are often called "Don't Give a Flip Pills" by the clients who take them because that's exactly how they feel. Their blood pressure is lowered (calcium influx blocked), pulse is decreased, and if they move too quickly they get dizzy. They are much happier being a couch potato and taking life easy. A few examples of the calcium channel blockers include **C**ardizem, **C**ardene, **P**rocardia, and **C**alan. Each of these common Calcium Channel Blockers have a **Ca** in them which makes it easy to remember! These medications should be administered with meals and milk. Some general undesirable effects of these medications include **constipation, bradycardia, peripheral edema, hypotension, dizziness, heart blocks, and worsening of CHF**.

*Remember–Calcium Channel blockers should **not** be given in clients who are in **congestive heart failure** or **cardiogenic shock** because they can decrease the heart rate too much.*

CALCIUM CHANNEL BLOCKERS

"DON'T GIVE A FLIP PILLS"

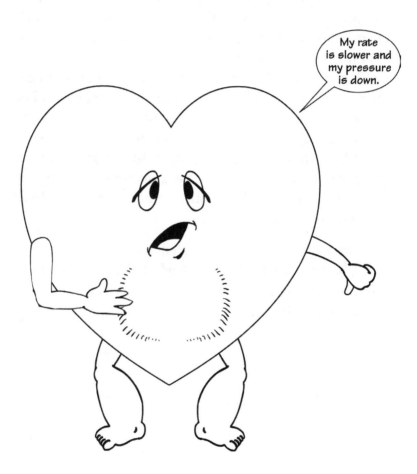

LOOP DIURETICS

Lou La Bell has been given a loop diuretic such as Lasix or Ethacrynate Sodium and is very **dizzy**. Her blood pressure has decreased too much after her excessive peeing. You would also feel as if you were spinning in a tube over the falls if you lost this much urine (volume). It may be very useful to teach her to get up slowly so she won't fall.

The life guard must blow his whistle in order to get her some assistance. She feels that the **ringing** in her ears just won't go away. **Dizziness** and **ringing** in the ears are major adverse reactions from loop diuretics.

A few other adverse reactions include: **hypokalemia, hypocalcemia (tetany), hyperglycemia**, and **hyperuricemia**. While aplastic anemia and agranulocytosis may occur, they are RARE!

Remember–Keep a close watch on blood pressure, potassium and calcium levels. Teach foods high in potassium and calcium. See ABC Fruit and Veggie Plate. Potassium supplements may be necessary.

LOU LA BELL

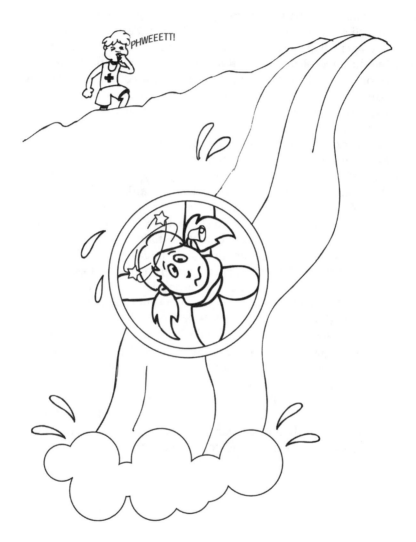

ATRIAL DYSRHYTHMIAS

If atrial fibrillation or atrial flutter occur greater than 48 hours in a client with normal cardiac function, diltiazem (Cardizem) is one agent that may be effective in controlling the **heart rate**. If the duration of the dysrhythmia is < 48 hours, consider the use of only one of the following agents for **converting the rhythm**: Amiodarone, Ibutilide, Flecainide, Propafenone, or Pocainamide. DC cardioversion. If the duration is > 48 hours or unknown, use antiarrhythmic agents with extreme caution. Avoid nonemergent cardioversion unless anticoagulation or clot precautions are taken. For specific management refer to *Handbook of Emergency Cardiovascular Care for Healthcare Providers* by American Heart Association. The management of delayed cardioversion and anticoagulation therapy are beyond the scope of this book.

In a client with an impaired heart (EF < 40% or CHF) and the AF > 48 hours duration, one of the following agents are recommended for controlling the **heart rate**: Digoxin, Diltiazem, Amiodarone. For this same client converting the AF in < 48 hours may be accomplished with Amiodarone. DC cardioversion. It the AF has persisted > 48 hours manage the anticoagulation and DC cardioversion. (*American Heart Association*)

Cardioversion may be indicated for heart rates >150 bpm with serious signs and symptoms related to tachycardia. Place the defibrillator/monitor in synchronized (sync) mode. The cardioversion may be painful due to the electric current going through the chest, therefore premedicate whenever possible.

Be prepared for the cardioversion to convert the rhythm to ventricular fibrillation. As our mothers always told us, too much of a good thing can be bad for us. Sometimes "stuff just happens!"

ATRIAL ACTIONS

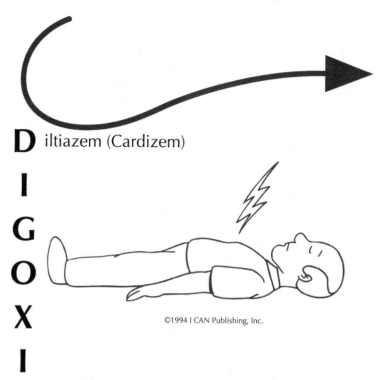

D iltiazem (Cardizem)

I

G

O

X

I

N ow lie 'em down for cardioversion

©1994 I CAN Publishing, Inc.

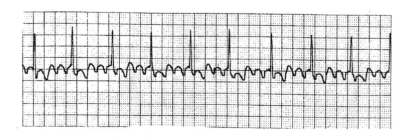

HEART BLOCKS

Heart Blocks are caused by a delay or interruption in electrical conduction between the atria and ventricles. This delay may be caused by cardiac disease process, Beta Blockers, and Calcium Channel Blockers. An electronic **Pacemaker** (transcutaneous pacing, TCP) is usually the preferred treatment for the more severe heart blocks. Drugs are often tried to correct this rhythm and **Atropine** is frequently the choice. Atropine blocks the vagus nerve impulses on the SA node causing an increased heart rate. **Ephinephrine** will also cause an increased heart rate.

According to current American Heart Association guidelines, if the client is exhibiting serious signs and symptoms due to the bradycardia, then the intervention sequence would be as outlined below.

Atropine – First Degree
Transcutaneous pacing if available – Second / Third Degree
Dopamine
Epinephrine

(For specific dosage, refer to *Handbook of Emergency Cardiovascular Care for Healthcare* Providers by American Heart Association)

If the client begins experiencing a Type II second-degree AV block or Third-degree AV block, prepare for transvenous pacer. If the symptoms develop, use the transcutaneous pacemaker until the transvenous pacer is placed.

*If a pacemaker is inserted, teach client how to monitor their pulse which is an indicator of pacemaker function. Teach symptoms of pacemaker dysfunction and pertinent detail regarding "power" failure in permanent pacemakers. Provide a safe environment by eliminating all possible electrical hazards. Instruct these clients to wear medical identification.

For additional specific algorithms refer to www.ACLS.net.
A special thank you to ACLS for outlining algorithms which are easy to remember!

HEART BLOCKS

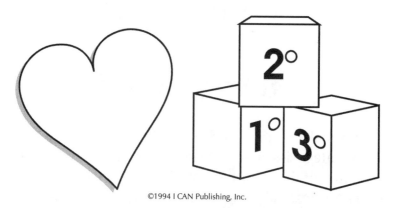

©1994 I CAN Publishing, Inc.

PACEMAKER

A
T   **A**
R   **T**
O   **R**
P   **I**
I
N
E

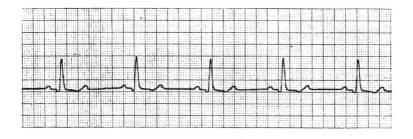

RESPIRATORY/ ACID BASE

BREATH SOUNDS

Normal breath sounds have been organized into three categories based upon the intensity, pitch, and duration of the inspiratory and expiratory phases.

The bronchial sounds are heard over the manubrium (if heard at all). The expiration sounds are longer than inspiration sounds. They are louder and higher in pitch. If these are auscultated anywhere other than the manubrium, they are considered to be abnormal and may indicate a complication with a lobar pneumonia.

The bronchovesicular sounds are heard often in the 1st and 2nd interspaces anteriorly and between the scapulae. The inspiratory and expiratory sounds are about equal in length. These sounds are intermediate. Differences in pitch and intensity are often more easily assessed during expiration. If bronchovesicular sounds are heard in other locations distant from what is listed above, then the air-filled lung may have been replaced by fluid or solid lung tissue.

The vesicular breath sounds may be auscultated over most of both lungs. Inspiratory sounds last longer than expiratory ones. Vesicular breath sounds are soft and low-pitched.

BREATH SOUNDS

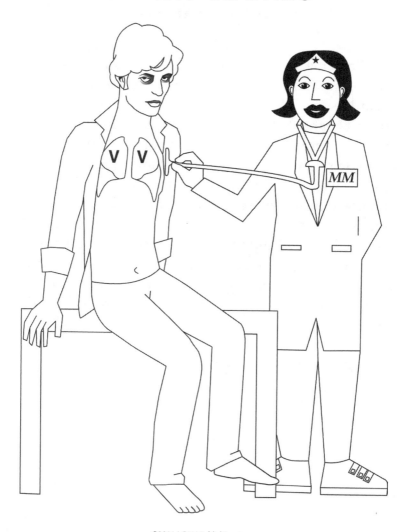

TRANSMITTED VOICE SOUNDS

When the lung is normal and filled with air, spoken words are indistinct and muffled. The spoken "ee" is heard as "ee." Whispered words are faint and indistinct if heard at all. They are normally accompanied by vesicular breath sounds and normal tactile fremitus.

When these sounds go through an airless lung such as in lobar pneumonia or toward the top of a large pleural effusion, these spoken sounds (99, ee, 1,2,3) are louder and clearer (bronchophony). The spoken "ee" is heard as "ay" and whispered words are louder and clearer (whispered pectoriloquy). These transmitted voice sounds are usually accompanied by bronchial or bronchovesicular breath sounds and increased tactile fremitus.

Note: Remember to end in "phony" (phonics)-to understand clarity. Increase in clarity = consolidation!!

TRANSMITTED VOICE SOUNDS

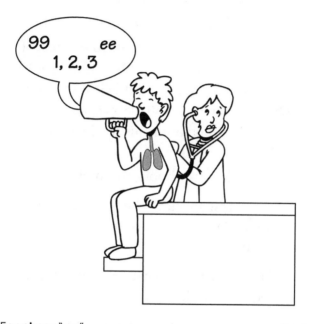

Ego**phony** "ee"	=	"ay" sound
Broncho**phony** "99"	=	clarity of sounds
Whispered Pectoriloquy	=	clarity of sounds
"whisper 99 or 1,2,3"		

↓

Clarity of Sounds

↓

CONSOLIDATION

DIAGNOSTICS
RESPIRATORY SYSTEM

Diagnostic testing is common in making respiratory diagnosis possible. A safe nurse will be able to answer these 3 questions about each of these Diagnostic Tests.

1. What should be completed prior to this test? (consent, teaching, allergies, holding meds or food).

2. What should happen during this test (positioning, anesthesia, invasive/noninvasive).

3. What should happen after this test? (reporting, monitoring)

MRI (Determine claustrophobia and metal)

Bronchoscopy, a test to view the airway, is invasive and requires sedation and consent. The biggest risk is pneumothorax.

Pulmonary Function Test, measures lung volume and does not require medication

VQ—Ventilation perfusion measures how well air reaches the lungs, requires consent and utilizes a radioisotope for imaging. Determine possible allergy to radioisotope used in the exam

PPD is an intradermal skin test for tuberculosis. Safe nurses must know how to determine positive/negative

Arterial Blood Gases used to measure oxygen and carbon dioxide in the blood to determine lung functioning. Safe nurses must know how to intervene after analyzing the results

DIAGNOSTICS
RESPIRATORY SYSTEM

Remember: Diagnostic exams can be hazardous to the health of our clients.

It is our mission to keep them safe.

The results of these exams are assessments that provide vital information for our critical thinking and clinical reasoning.

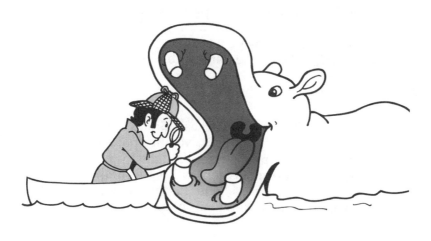

©2008 I CAN Publishing, Inc.

PULMONARY EDEMA

This condition is a result of too much fluid in the lung, both in the interstitial and in the alveolar spaces. Pulmonary edema results from severe impairment of the left heart function. MAD DOG COMES TO THE RESCUE!

M **MORPHINE** will decrease preload, allowing blood to pool in the extremities. As a result, the heart will not work as hard. A major problem is anxiety, due to feeling they are drowning in their secretions. Although morphine will decrease the anxiety, monitor for potential respiratory depression.

A **AMINOPHYLLINE** will decrease shortness of breath by expanding the bronchi. (Refer to Aminophylline Toxicity for more specific information.)

D **DIGOXIN** slows heart rate by increasing cardiac output. Hold med if apical heart rate below 60. Therapeutic level is 0.6–2.0 mg/ml; above 2.0 mg/ml is toxic. Signs of toxicity are anorexia, nausea, vomiting, headache, fatigue, bradycardia and photophobia.

D **DIURETICS**, especially Lasix dump the fluid overload through the kidneys. Monitor potassium level. Hypokalemia precipitates digitalis toxicity. (Therapeutic level of potassium is 3.5–5.0 mEq/L.) Daily weight will help evaluate the fluid loss along with an accurate intake and output record.

O **OXYGEN** is given to saturate red blood cells and provide more oxygen to the tissues. Oxygen is usually given via nasal cannula.

G **GASES** are evaluated to maintain pH, PO_2 and PCO_2 within appropriate limits. (Refer to **ACID-BASE**.)

PULMONARY EDEMA

M orphine

A minophylline

D igoxin

D iuretics

O xygen

G ases

ACID-BASE

Draw a line down the middle of the right page. At the top of the left column put the numbers 7.35. At the top of the right column put 7.45. The normal blood pH should stay between these numbers. A pH below 7.35 indicates acidosis. A pH above 7.45 indicates alkalosis. Under 7.35 write CO_2 (body turns carbon dioxide to carbonic acid). Under 7.45 write HCO_3. Under HCO_3 write HCO_3 again and again. If we had enough paper we would write HCO_3 20 times because normal ratio of HCO_3 to pCO_2 is 20:1. The objective is to keep the pH between 7.35 and 7.45 which is done with buffer systems.

COLOR the van red. The red van represents the blood buffer system. Imagine the van driving through the arteries and veins of your body. When the pH gets below 7.35 (acidosis) the back van door opens, out jumps 20 little bicarbs, neutralizes the acid and gets back in the van to drive off! If the ph gets above 7.45 (alkalosis) the front van door opens, big powerful CO_2 jumps out, neutralizes and gets back in to drive off. This blood buffer is the first buffer system to respond to pH variations. The lungs follow by adjusting the res-pirations to regulate the CO_2. The third buffer system that helps maintain the pH are the kidneys.

ACID-BASE

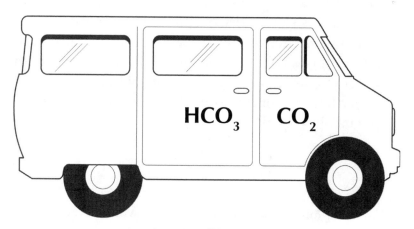

ACID-BASE STATUS

To determine acid-base status (respiratory or metabolic), picture yourself in Rome. You are on a playground with Phonetia (pH), Carbo (HCO_3), and Paco (pCO_2).

Phonetia and Paco hop on the see-saw and begin to play. Up and down, up and down. When the pH and pCO_2 are in opposite directions from "normal," the status is respiratory (respiratory = opposite).

Phonetia tires of playing with Paco and runs off to join Carbo who is on a swing. Both go up and both go down, always together. When pH and HCO_3 are either both up or both down, the status is metabolic (metabolic=equal).

pH > 7.45 = alkalosis
pH < 7.35 = acidosis

(Turn page for COMPENSATORY MECHANISMS).

Reprinted with permission from Creative Educators, Jefferson, LA

ACID-BASE STATUS

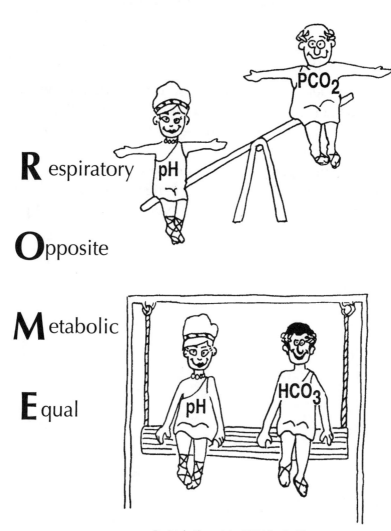

Respiratory

Opposite

Metabolic

Equal

Reprinted with permission ©1994 Creative Educators

COMPENSATORY MECHANISMS

(This will make more sense to you if you first refer to ACID-BASE STATUS.)

Compensation occurs in respiratory situations when Carbo gets mad at Phonetia for playing with Paco and hops on Paco's side of the see-saw! Imagine all three on the same see-saw.

Compensation occurs in metabolic situations when Paco decides to crash the swinging twosome and hops on with Phonetia and Carbo. Now all go up or all go down.

Reprinted with permission from Creative Educators, Jefferson, LA

COMPENSATORY MECHANISMS

Respiratory

Metabolic

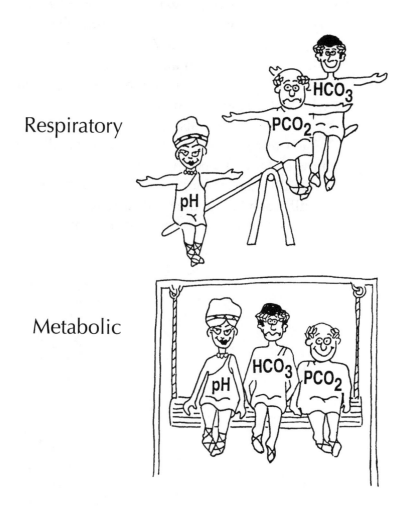

ACID-BASE

This referee is calling the shots in Acid-Base. He will help you remember if **ACID** or **BASE** is lost. Think, **A**bove the waist **A**cid is lost. **B**elow the waist **B**ase is lost. The stomach, above the waist, contains HCl (H+ is an acid). HCl acid is lost during vomiting or when the client has a nasogastric tube. As a result, the client may develop a problem with alkalosis. When a client is hyperventilating, he increases the loss of carbon dioxide which also results in alkalosis.

The bowel below the waist contains alkaline substances which are lost during diarrhea. If alkali are lost, then the client may become acidotic.

There's a BIG exception here! Deep, prolonged vomiting will reach below the waist and lose alkaline intestinal juices resulting in a ketoacidotic state.

CALLING THE SHOTS
IN ACID VS. BASE

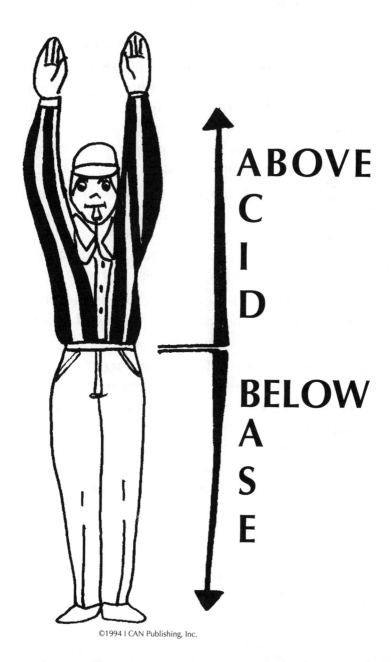

A
C
I
D

ABOVE

BELOW

B
A
S
E

©1994 I CAN Publishing, Inc.

SHOCK

When you think about the pathophysiology of shock, the classifications (except cardiogenic) have the common bond of decreased venous return (DVR).

HYPOVOLEMIC SHOCK (Hemorrhagic)–If an arm is cut off, that blood is certainly not returning to the heart. DVR! Another example of hypovolemic shock is the guy decides to roof his house on the 4th of July, and sweats out his volume, resulting in dehydration. Less blood to pump = DVR!

NEUROGENIC SHOCK–A severed spinal cord from a gunshot wound or fall allows blood to pool. Nerves have been cut; there is less venous constriction due to absent nerve stimulation. Spinal anesthesia and barbiturate overdose will cause the same response.

SEPTIC SHOCK (toxic)–An overwhelming infection; generally gram negative organisms will cause a dilation of the blood vessels resulting in a DVR.

VASOGENIC SHOCK (anaphylactic)–A DVR results from an antigen-antibody reaction with release of histamine. Blood that pools causes DVR! Less blood to pump = DVR!

(Refer to **Shock Interventions**.)

In contrast, CARDIOGENIC SHOCK is volume overload NOT volume deficit.

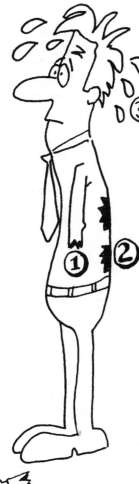

Shock is Decreased Venous Return

except Cardiogenic

HELP STAMP OUT SHOCK

S   **SOLUTIONS** add volume and will increase venous return. Increase the rate. A combination of fluids, blood and plasma expanders (dextran, plasma and albumin) are commonly used. Watch for I.V.s with meds in them. We wouldn't want to turn up the I.V. rate of Pitocin!

H   **HEMODYNAMICS** are a way to measure potential shock and evaluate interventions. CVP–(normal is a lucky 7) low CVP means DVR, (decreased venous return) or fluid deficit. Elevated CVP means fluid overload as seen in cardiogenic shock. Low BP reading is one parameter that spells trouble.

Monitor it every few minutes. As meds are given to increase the BP, it may come up quickly.

EARLY CHANGES	LATE CHANGES
Anxious	Coma
Heart rate elevated	Heart rate elevated and weak
Respirations elevated and deep	Respirations elevated and shallow
Skin cool, moist	Skin cold, clammy
Blood pressure no change	Blood pressure decreased
Normal skin color	Pale skin color

O   **OXYGEN** will saturate those red blood cells and decrease tissue starvation.

C   **CHECK** the skin which is often cold and clammy.

K   **KICK** up those feet and legs! There's a lot of blood volume in those legs. Elevate them and let gravity help increase venous return. Don't put the head down. Trendelenburg position may increase cranial pressure, ocular pressure and pressure on the diaphragm.

HELP STAMP OUT SHOCK

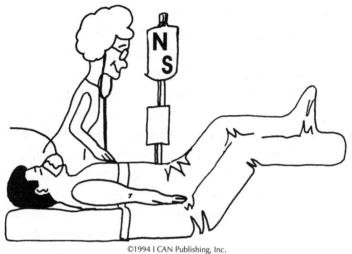

©1994 I CAN Publishing, Inc.

Solutions

Hemodynamic changes

Oxygen

Checking

Kick 'em up

LUNG SOUNDS

Just breathing in and out makes a normal lung sound that can be heard with a stethoscope. Listen to both sides of the chest because the right side can have clear lung sounds while the left side can have "rales," "wheezes" or some adventitious breath sounds. Listen to the anterior (front) and posterior (back) sounds. How do we know if we hear rales? Rales, sounding like Rice Krispies doing "snap, crackle and pop," are most commonly heard around alveolar sacs more distal to the bronchial tubes. Rales have also been compared to the fizzling of a carbonated drink and are usually heard midway through the inspiratory phase. Wheezes are most often found over the midline or bronchi indicating constriction. Wheezes are continuous sounds, although they are heard more on expiration. Imagine hearing a whistle blow! This is similar to a wheeze.

The bottom line is that breath sounds should be clear and air should be heard moving on both inspiration and expiration. The key is to know what the normal is, so you can detect a difference.

ABNORMAL LUNG SOUNDS

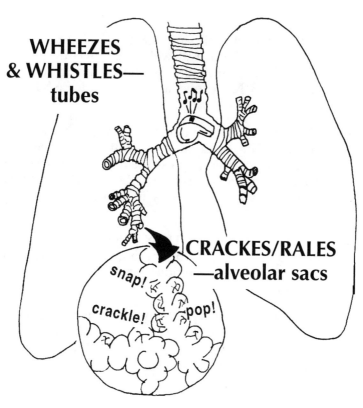

©1994 I CAN Publishing, Inc.

COPD

Chronic Obstructive Pulmonary Disease is referred to as emphysema. A major risk factor is cigarette smoking.

C **COUGH** is chronic and nonproductive making it hard to breathe or rest well. A chest x-ray is often ordered to confirm the diagnosis and to look for pneumonia. Nope, one does not have to be NPO for a chest x-ray.

O **OXYGEN** starvation demands oxygen. A good rule of thumb for the O_2 flow is 2-4 liters. High concentrations of oxygen depress the drive to breathe and cause respiratory distress. ABG's (arterial blood gases) are an excellent way to measure what's happening.

P **PULMONARY FUNCTION TEST** shows a decrease in lung function possibly calling for postural drainage to reduce secretions and increase oxygen exchange.

D **DON'T SMOKE** is probably excellent advice. Emotional support usually helps; nagging doesn't. Drugs and other stuff often given for COPD are included on the next page.

CHRONIC OBSTRUCTIVE PULMONARY DISEASE

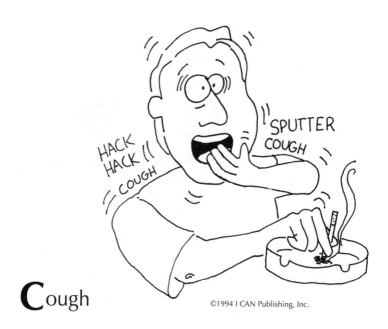

©1994 I CAN Publishing, Inc.

Cough

Oxygen and ABG's

Pulmonary function and postural drainage

Don't smoke

INTERVENTIONS FOR COPD (CHRONIC OBSTRUCTIVE PULMONARY DISEASE)

Since our primary objective for these clients is to enhance oxygen exchange, it makes sense to look at these medicines around the ABC's.

A   **ANTI-INFLAMMATORY (CORTICOSTEROIDS)** May be used to decrease inflammation. Example: Betamethasone *(Remember: Excellent oral hygiene to prevent candida infections from corticosteroids).*

B   **BRONCHODILATORS**–Epinephrine (adrenalin) is also used to relax smooth muscle of bronchials. Do not use if client has hypertension or cardiac arrhythmias. Example: Albuterol.

C   **CHEST PHYSIOTHERAPY**–Help remove secretions from the lungs. (Refer to Postural Drainage.)

D   **DELIVER OXYGEN AT 2 LITERS**–High concentrations of oxygen would eliminate the client's hypoxic drive and cause respiratory distress.

E   **EXPECTORANTS**–These will assist in decreasing the viscosity of the mucous.

F   **FORCE FLUIDS**–Fluids will facilitate the removal of secretions.

INTERVENTIONS FOR COPD
(A B C'S)

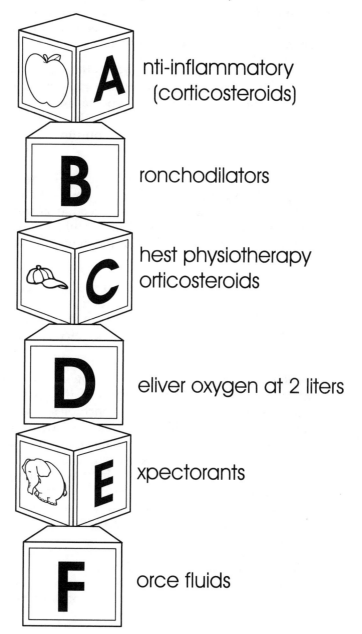

A nti-inflammatory (corticosteroids)

B ronchodilators

C hest physiotherapy orticosteroids

D eliver oxygen at 2 liters

E xpectorants

F orce fluids

©1994 I CAN

ASTHMA

INFL A MMATION–Asthma is a chronic inflammatory process that produces mucosal edema, mucus secretion, and airway inflammation.

S SYMPTOMS–Wheezing, chest tightness, shortness of breath, cough. Use of accessory muscles in breathing. Symptoms of hypoxia and cyanosis occur late. Increased anxiety, restlessness, and exercise intolerance. Excessive sputum production.

T TREATMENT-includes beta$_2$ adrenergic medications by nebulizer or metered dose inhalers. Epinephrine, antibiotics (if an infection is present), broncho-dilators, expectorants. Inhalation of steroids to prevent edema. Supplemental oxygen for hypoxemia.

IN H ALERS- Inhalation of steroids to prevent edema. Beta$_2$-Adrenergic Agonists stimulate beta receptors in the lung, relax bronchial smooth muscle, increase vital capacity, and decrease airway resistance.

M MECHANISMS–Intermittent narrowing of the airway is caused by constriction of the smooth muscles of the bronchi and bronchioles. Excessive mucus production and mucosal edema of the respiratory tract are other mechanisms that contribute to asthma. Constriction of smooth muscle results in a significant increased airway resistance, resulting in trapped air in the lung. Emotional factors are also known to play an important role in precipitating an asthmatic attack for the child.

A AVOID ALLERGENS–Educate client regarding the importance of avoiding allergens that have been identified as precipitating factors resulting in an asthmatic attack.

ASTHMA

infl **A**mmation

Symptoms

Treatment

in**H**alers

Mechanisms

Avoidance

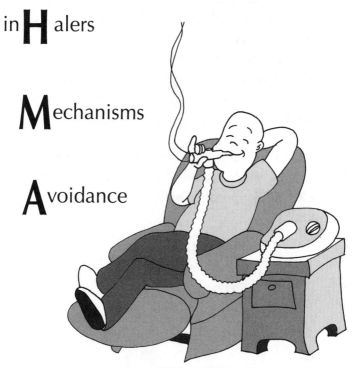

BETA$_2$-ADRENERGIC AGONISTS

MAX AIR, our friend on the next page, is holding several balloons to assist you in remembering some key points with these medications. Notice the balloons on the left are the clinical outcomes we expect from **MAX AIR**. Beta$_2$-Adrenergic Agonists stimulate the beta receptors in the lung, resulting in the relaxation of bronchial smooth muscles. This action results in an increased vital capacity which allows clients to breathe easier, resulting in the ability to blow up balloons.

Unfortunately, there are some undesirable effects that may occur while taking these medications. The balloons on the right will help you remember some key points. Tachycardia, irregular heart beat, hypertension, or cardiac dysrhythmias may occur. In addition to cardiac irregularities, other undesirable effects that may occur include nervousness, tremors, restlessness, insomnia, headache; nausea, or vomiting.

NOTE: For specific details about these drugs refer to *Pharmacology Made Insanely Easy* by Loretta Manning and Sylvia Rayfield. Specific details for ordering are in the back of this book.

BETA₂-ADRENERGIC AGONISTS

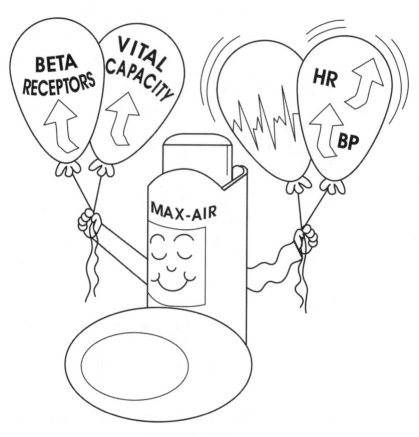

CYSTIC FIBROSIS

This little guy is a "**SICKER KID.**" His disease is inherited from an autosomal recessive trait. The exocrine glands that normally produce the enzymes lipase (digests fats), trypsin (digests protein) and amylase (digests starches) are not functioning normally. He's doing without a good part of his nutrition (about 40% of his food gets ingested). The other issue is that cystic fibrosis causes these enzymes to become so tenacious that they cause other problems. Organs affected by this disease include the lungs, pancreas, GI tract, and liver. "**Sicker Kid**" will assist you in remembering the major concepts in cystic fibrosis.

S   **STEATORRHEA** (fat in stool) smelly stools with increased amount.

    SWEAT TEST indicating high salt content may be diagnostic. Adequate salt intake is important.

I   **ILEUS-MECONIUM** may be present in newborns. The small intestine is blocked with thick mucous causing symptoms of intestinal obstruction.

C   **CONSTANT HUNGER** because of poor food absorption.

K   **VITAMINS K, A, D, E** (fat soluble) may be supplemented.

E   **ENZYME (pancreatic) REPLACEMENT** is mandatory. Administer prior to meals and snacks.

R   **REDUCE** dietary fat. Use **low fat** milk.

K   **KEEP CALORIES UP**. Use **simple sugars** as a source of energy.

I   **INFECTION** may be a way of life, especially respiratory infections due to pulmonary congestion. Administer oxygen and IV fluids to keep secretions thin.

D   **DRINK PLENTY OF FLUIDS** to prevent dehydration and to keep mucous thin. DIET high in calorie, high protein, fats as tolerated or decreased, and increase salt intake.

CYSTIC FIBROSIS

S teatorrhea
weat test

I leus-meconium

C onstant hunger

K vitamins

E nzyme replacement

R educe fat

K eep calories up

I nfection

D rink plenty of fluids

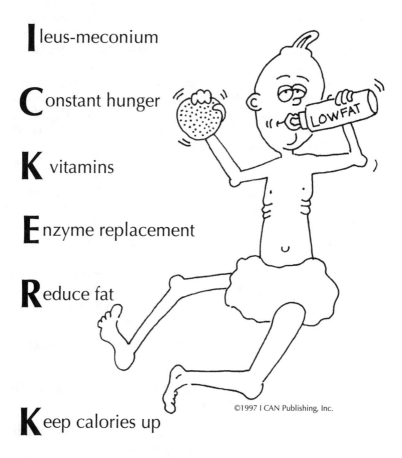

©1997 I CAN Publishing, Inc.

VENTILATOR CARE

This poor guy has found himself on a ventilator. To accurately evaluate the effectiveness of the vent, closely **VIEW** the client's **ARTERIAL BLOOD GASES**. Pressure should be maintained at the puncture site for a minimum of 5 minutes. After changing any ventilatory settings or suctioning the client, wait for 30 minutes to draw the ABG's. After procedures, carefully evaluate client's vital signs, pulse oximetry, color, etc., and check that **VENT** alarms are on. To determine the adequacy of air exchange, **EVALUATE** the **BREATH SOUNDS**. Look for equal chest movement, client's color and respirations. Calmly explain equipment and alarms to both the client and family. Ventilators are such a scary proposition that people become stressed. **NOTICE GI COMPLICATIONS** from potential **STRESS ULCERS**. The majority of clients will require a H_2 Histamine Antagonist.

The nurse must **TAKE NOTICE OF PRESSURE ALARMS** on the ventilator. An easy way to remember this information is that if the low alarm goes off, the priority of care is to check for a leak. To assist you in remembering this, *note there is a l in* **low** *and a l in* **leak**. If the high pressure alarm goes off, *remember* **high** *rhymes with* **dry**. The client may need suctioning or there may be water in the ventilator tubes. The tubes or client needs to dry out.

Here is a quick way to prioritize nursing actions when the ventilator alarm goes off. Do you remember the old saying, "Katie BARS the door"? Think about that when the ventilator alarm goes off and "**BARS**" will give you your priorities.

B   Bag the client because the ventilator is not working. He can't breathe!

A   Assess for lung sounds. This will let you know if the client can breathe on his own.

R   Repair the vent. Faulty equipment is not an excuse for inappropriate nursing action.

S   Secretions must drain. Keep HOB elevated at 30 to 45 degrees.

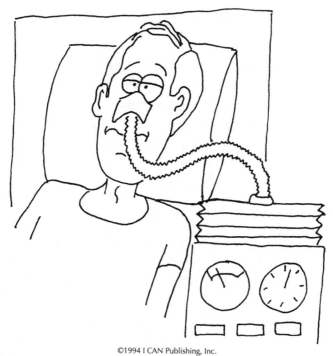

©1994 I CAN Publishing, Inc.

View ABG's

Evaluate breath sounds

Notice G.I. complications (stress ulcer)

Take notice of pressure alarms

TUBERCULOSIS

INA has the typical signs and symptoms of tuberculosis including fatigue, weight loss, anorexia, chronic productive cough, night sweats, and hemoptysis (advanced stage). In order to help the *mycobacterium tuberculosis* rise out of her, there are several medications which may be prescribed. "**RISE**" will assist in remembering these medications.

R   **RIFAMPIN**–This medication is most often prescribed with isoniazid (INH). The secretions (sweat, urine) may turn orange. Hepatitis may be a complication, especially in alcoholics. Rifampin should be administered once daily on an empty stomach.

I   **ISONIAZID (INH)**–This is the primary medication used in prophylactic treatment of tuberculosis. Adverse reactions include hepatitis, and/or hepatotoxicity. Peripheral neuropathies can be prevented by pretreating with pyridoxine (vitamin B6). INH should be administered once daily on an empty stomach.

S   **STREPTOMYCIN**–Two major adverse effects from this medication are ototoxicity and nephrotoxicity. Due to the susceptibility to cranial nerve VIII, this medication is generally avoided in the elderly. Use it with caution if clients have renal disease. Hearing must be evaluated frequently. Streptomycin may not be given po.

E   **ETHAMBUTOL**–This medication is frequently administered with rifampin and INH. Assess vision prior to therapy to identify side effects of optic neuritis which may result in loss of central vision from this medication. Ethambutol should be administered once daily with food or meals to decrease gastric irritation.

INA TUBERCULOSIS

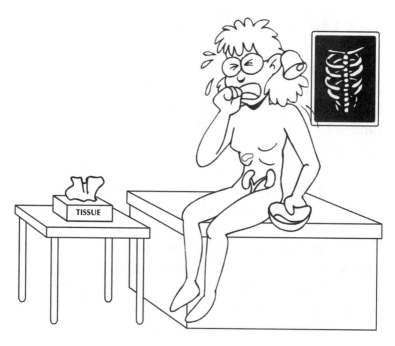

©1997 I CAN Publishing, Inc.

FLUID VOLUME / RENAL SYSTEM

FLUID VOLUME STATUS

The arrow indicates that fluid (plasma) volume decreases during dehydration. This will cause an increase in the sodium blood level above the normal range of 135-145 meq/L. The hematocrit will also rise (above 45%) due to the same principle.

The opposite occurs during pregnancy. Due to increased fluid (plasma) levels, the hematocrit and the serum sodium levels decrease. This dilution of the red blood cells is referred to as pseudoanemia. Evaluation of the serum sodium and hematocrit levels are excellent indicators of the fluid volume status. Several important nursing interventions for these clients include: daily weights, intake and output records, specific gravity evaluation of the urine, assessing the skin turgor, and lips and mucous membranes. An important assessment for infants regarding their fluid status is to observe if the fontanels are depressed or bulging.

This is an excellent tool to assist you in remembering the concept of the fluid volume status.

Assessment for fluid volume may be determined by blood work.
Normal sodium blood level 135-145 meq/L
Normal Potassium level 3.5-5 meq/L
Normal Hemoglobin ranges with age-adults 12-14 gm/dl
Normal Red Cell Count adult women 4.2-5.4, men 4.7-6.1 million/uL
Or
Skin Tugor, lips, mucous membranes, daily weights

FLUID VOLUME STATUS

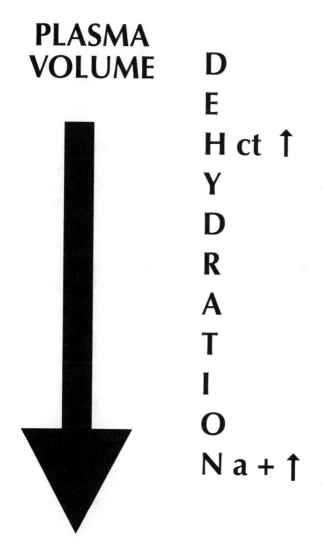

PLASMA VOLUME

D
E
H ct ↑
Y
D
R
A
T
I
O
N a + ↑

FLUID SHIFTS

Fluid shifts are easier to figure out if you remember this nursery rhyme:

"Mary had a little lamb and everywhere Mary went, the lamb was sure to go." Mary is salt (NaCl), and the lamb is water. Everywhere salt goes, water follows.

You may be asking yourself, how does this fit in with my nursing care? Frequently, we need to do health teaching for clients who are taking certain medications. The group that comes to our mind are the thiazides. Would we want these individuals eating a high sodium diet? Of course not! That would defeat the purpose for these diuretics.

Diuretics are given to remove fluid from the body. If we increase the sodium intake for these clients, they will continue to retain fluid. Everywhere salt (NaCl) goes, water follows.

FLUID SHIFTS

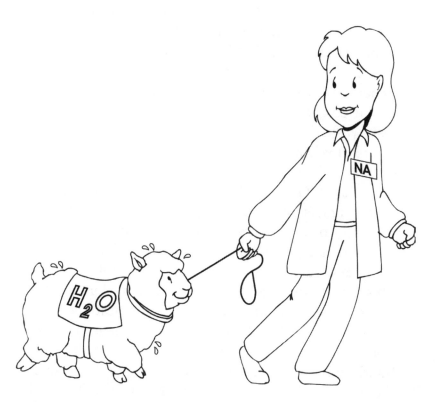

©1994 I CAN Publishing, Inc.

"Mary had a little lamb and everywhere Mary went the lamb was sure to go."

RENAL PATHOLOGY

This system can be quite simple when you compare it to a water faucet and pitcher as we have on the image page. In the normal (healthy) faucet, the flow is great. There is no obstruction, and the filter is fine.

Notice in the **PRERENAL** diagram, there is decrease in the flow of water (urine). There is faucet (renal) ischemia–a decrease in the water pressure. Have you ever tried getting hot water out of the faucet while the dish washer is on? This can occur in the renal system from hemorrhage, shock, burns or decreased cardiac output.

In the **INTRARENAL** diagram, there is decreased output and some WBC's and protein which do not normally belong in the urine. This is due to kidney tissue pathology. In the faucet, it is as if someone came along and cut an opening in the filter on the spicket. This may be from glomerulonephritis, pyelonephritis, severe crushing injury, chemicals or medications.

In the **POSTRENAL** diagram, there is an obstruction in the water flow. This could be from the lime build up in the system which is causing a decrease in the free fluid. This is exactly what happens in the renal system. Some examples are: urinary calculi, benign prostatic hypertrophy (BPH) and cancer.

Remember to check renal function tests, BUN 10–20, creatinine .5–1.5. As the renal function decreases, these values will increase.

RENAL PATHOLOGY

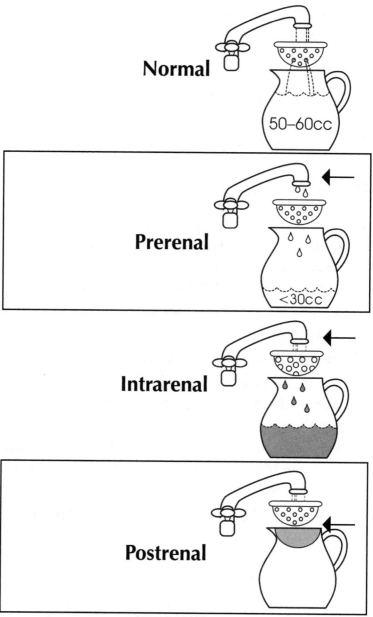

Normal

50–60cc

Prerenal

<30cc

Intrarenal

Postrenal

DIAGNOSTICS RENAL SYSTEM

Diagnostic testing is common in making renal diagnosis possible. A safe nurse will be able to answer these 3 questions about each of these Diagnostic Tests.

1. What should be completed prior to this test (consent, teaching, allergies, holding meds or food)?
2. What should happen during this test (positioning, anesthesia, invasive/noninvasive)?
3. What should happen after this test (reporting, monitoring)?

Specific Gravity of Urine – shows concentrating/diluting ability of kidney. Some examples (reduced sg = excess fluid intake, diabetes mellitus or insipidus), (raised sg = dehydration, sweating, congestive heart failure, renal stenosis, liver disease). Normal 1.001-1.030 g/ml.

KUB – xray of abdominal structures includes kidneys and bladder. Noninvasive.

Bladder Scan – noninvasive ultrasound

IVP – intravenous pyleogram of the kidney. Utilizes dye. Determine allergy to iodine (shrimp, seafood).

Cystoscopy examines the bladder and uretha, usually under mind anesthesia/consent needed. Drink lots of water.

CT guided renal biopsy for renal masses. Anesthesia often local.

DIAGNOSTICS RENAL SYSTEM

Remember: Diagnostic exams can be hazardous to the health of our clients.

It is our mission to keep them safe.

The results of these exams are assessments that provide vital information for our critical thinking and clinical reasoning.

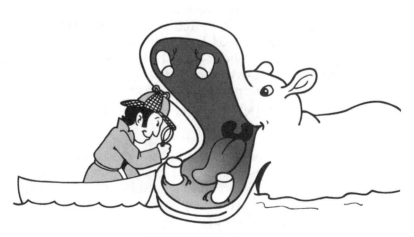

BURNS

Berny has been in a fire, and as you can see, he is wrapped up like a mummy. Berny BURNS will help us learn burn care.

B   **BREATHING**–Keep airway open. Facial burns, singed nasal hair, hoarseness, sooty sputum, bloody sputum, and labored respirations indicate TROUBLE!

BODY IMAGE–Assist Berny in coping by encouraging expression of thoughts and feelings.

U   **URINE OUTPUT**–In an adult, urine output should be 30 to 70 cc per hour, in the child 20 to 50 cc per hour, and in the infant 10 to 20 cc per hour. Watch the K+ to keep it between 3.5–5.0 mEq/L. Keep the CVP around 12 cm water pressure.

R   **RESUSCITATION OF FLUID**–Salt and electrolyte solutions are essential over the first 24 hours. Maintain BP at 90 to 100 systolic. One-half of the fluid for the first 24 hours should be administered over the first 8-hour period, then the remainder is administered over the next 16 hours. First 24-hour calculation starts at the time of injury.

RULE OF NINE–Used for adults to determine burn surface area.

N   **NUTRITION**–Protein and calories are components of the diet. Supplemental gastric tube feedings or hyperalimentation may be used in clients with large burned areas. Daily weights will assist in evaluating the nutritional needs.

S   **SHOCK**–Watch the BP, CVP and renal function.

SILVADENE–For infection.

REMEMBER THESE PEOPLE ARE AFRAID
AND NEED SUPPORT!

BURNS

B reathing
B ody image

U rine output

R ule of nine
R esuscitation of fluid

N utrition

S hock
S ilvadene

MEN & WOMEN'S CARE / CANCER

BENIGN PROSTATE HYPERTROPHY

The poor guy who has his "tubes" squeezed tightly due to an enlarged prostate gland will likely find himself going to surgery for a transurethral resection of the prostate (TURP). Prostatic tissue is removed through a resectoscope, so the urethra can once again pass urine easily.

When the guy comes back from surgery, he will likely have a triple lumen tube in his bladder to maintain continuous bladder irrigation (CBI) or Murphy drip. The **TUBE** will provide for **URINARY OUTPUT**, but it will contain bright **RED DRAINAGE**. If you see pieces of clots in the tube, it's time to increase the CBI to wash out the clots. Retained blood **CLOTS** may cause hemorrhage and we do not want that to happen! Unfortunately **CLOTS** may also cause bladder **SPASMS** that hurt. Belladonna and opium suppositories (B&O) are often ordered to help relieve the spasms. If the client complains of pain, evaluate the urinary drainage and make sure the catheter is patent.

Obstructions most commonly occur in the initial 24 hours due to clots in the bladder. Overdistention of the bladder can precipitate hemorrhage as well as bladder spasms.

TURPS

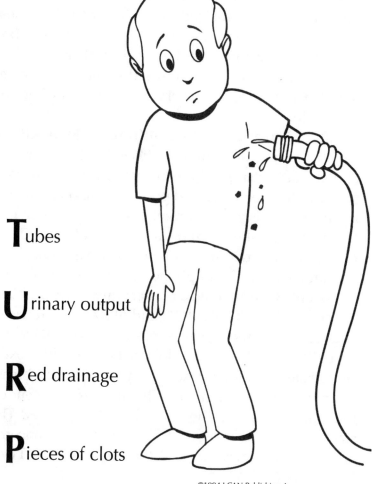

Tubes

Urinary output

Red drainage

Pieces of clots

©1994 I CAN Publishing, Inc.

Spasms

CARE OF CLIENT AFTER MASTECTOMY

Have you ever had a chicken without a breast? Well, this may be a first for you. Meet "Ester the breastless chicken." Ester had a mastectomy due to cancer. She has a family history with both her mother and sister having breast cancer. She refused to have the recommended mammogram every 1 to 2 years after she turned 40.

After her mastectomy, no **BLOOD PRESSURES** or lab sticks were done on the affected side. She maintained the affected side in an **ELEVATED** position. Each joint was to be elevated and positioned higher than the more proximal joint to promote drainage. Ester met some wonderful women from **REACH FOR RECOVERY** who provided her with support. She was given pamphlets to read and phone numbers of some contact people who also had a mastectomy. After they left, she started her **EXTENSION** and **FLEXION** exercises. Squeezing a ball is a great exercise. **ABDUCTION** and **EXTERNAL** rotation should not be the initial exercises. Ester was taught how to do a SBE (self breast examination) once a month. The nurse recommended that she do it while she was taking her shower. The staff encouraged Ester to discuss her fears, concerns and anxieties in order **TO PROMOTE A POSITIVE SELF-IMAGE**.

CARE OF CLIENT
AFTER MASTECTOMY

B P—not on affected side

R each for Recovery

E levate affected side
xtension and flexion
exercises—initially
(squeeze a ball)

A bduction and external rotation
should not be initial exercise

©1994 I CAN Publishing, Inc.

S B E—once a month—about one
week after period

T o promote a positive self-image

MENOPAUSE

MINNIE wakes up nights, throwing off those covers and finding herself wet with sweat from a hot flash. She reaches for her comfort measures with one hand since it will help control these night sweats and her heart shaped fan with the other. Her fan will cool her down, and it is heart shaped because during this time in her life she may wear her heart on her sleeve. She can be very sensitive and moody during menopause and small comments hurt her feelings. The estrogen will also improve Minnie's lipid profile and will decrease risks to her heart. (Refer to Josephine Bone-A-Part for more detail regarding estrogen.)

Vaginal BLEEDING seems to increase at menstrual period times and MINNIE must always be prepared with "supplies" because she can never tell when that period will show up. Excessive bleeding leads to ANEMIA and now she's got to take iron along with her other drugs, herbs and teas that reduce these "NO FUN symptoms."

Remember–This "PAUSE" is not a brief time in one's life and cannot be fixed quickly. Often symptoms persist for 3+ years!

MINNIE PAUSE

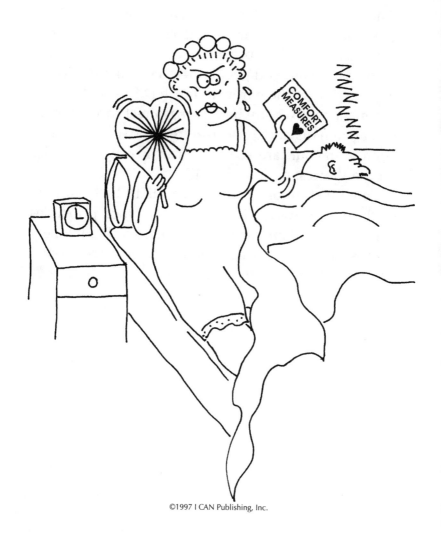

SAFETY WITH RADIUM IMPLANTS

"How do you feel today" is adopted from Sue Crow's book *Asepsis, The Right Touch*, an excellent down to earth book on infection control. Let's assume that the character in the bed has a radium implant.

We want to plan our nursing care from afar! When you are in very close proximity to the client who has a radium implant, you get almost as much radiation as they do. Talk to them from as much DISTANCE as you can manage. Except when giving direct care, attempt to maintain distance of six feet from the source of radiation. Plan your care, so that you are in close proximity for the shortest period of TIME.

Some institutions provide lead SHIELDING; generally not necessary if time and distance principles are observed. Remember, these clients will get lonely because they are on bedrest and can't leave their room. *Be sure they can reach the telephone and the call light!*

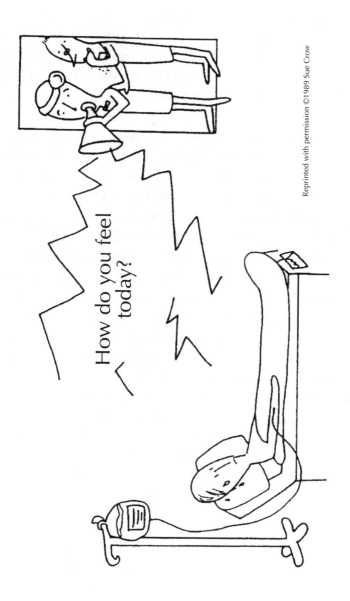

EXTERNAL RADIATION

Sammy Shade is receiving external radiation for cancer. This source of radiation is directed toward the area of the tumor and draining lymphatics. He is likely to experience **SEVERE NAUSEA AND VOMITING, HEMATURIA** *and* **DIARRHEA**. Meticulous oral hygiene is important to decrease complications associated with vomiting. Antidiarrheal medications, low residue, high protein and a bland diet will decrease complications of diarrhea. Notice, Sammy has no hair on his head, very little on his face and probably none in his pubic area. Sammy will need help to cope with changes in his body image due to **ALOPECIA**. He may decide to wear a wig or turban. Sammy needs to pat, not rub, hair dry after shampooing to avoid excessive handling of brittle hair. Ice packs to the scalp may reduce hair loss. **ANEMIA** is a common side effect of therapy. Maintain adequate rest in between scheduled activities. Evaluate Sammy for signs of hypoxia. Encourage a diet high in protein, vitamins and iron. Assess for signs of infection and bleeding. External radiation is prone to **DRY THE SKIN** particularly **EVALUATE** the site of radiation. This site may remain photophobic, so let's advise Sammy to remain in the **SHADE**.

EXTERNAL RADIATION

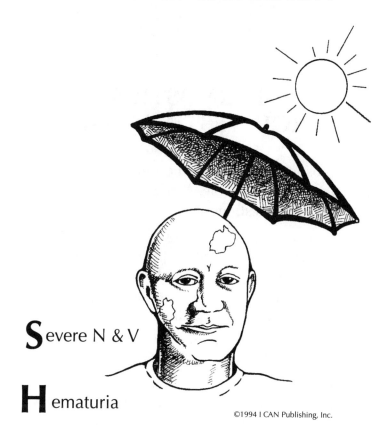

©1994 I CAN Publishing, Inc.

Severe N & V

Hematuria

A lopecia
nemia

D iarrhea

E valuate skin for redness/dryness

GASTROINTESTINAL SYSTEM

DIAGNOSTICS
GASTROINTESTINAL SYSTEM

Diagnostic testing is common in making gastrointestinal diagnosis possible. A safe nurse will be able to answer these 3 questions about each of these Diagnostic Tests.

1. What should be completed prior to this test (consent, teaching, allergies, holding meds or food)?
2. What should happen during this test (positioning, anesthesia, invasive/noninvasive)?
3. What should happen after this test (reporting, monitoring)?

X-Ray, noninvasive

The following tests are NO fun and include prep:

Upper GI, Barium Swallow, (NPO). Biopsy may be done.

Lower GI and Colonoscopy (extensive bowel cleansing). Biopsy may be done with either of these.

Colonoscopy utilizes conscious sedation and consent.

Endoscopy often utilizes conscious sedation and consent. Used to visualize stomach and duodenum growths, abnormalities, and bleeding. NPO, hold some medications.

CT guided Liver Biopsy to obtain a small piece of the liver for diagnosis. Often done under local anesthesia

DIAGNOSTICS
GASTROINTESTINAL SYSTEM

Remember: Diagnostic exams can be hazardous to the health of our clients.

It is our mission to keep them safe.

The results of these exams are assessments that provide vital information for our critical thinking and clinical reasoning.

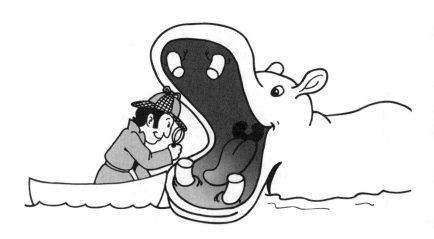

PEPTIC ULCER DISEASE

Old **PUD** is a fine specimen of a man. He's standing there tapping his foot waiting impatiently on that bus, smoking his cigarette with a vengeance and checking to see if it's time for another NSAID (Nonsteroidal Anti-inflammatory drugs may cause GI bleeding). Just the kind of behavior that might precipitate peptic ulcer disease. When you think ulcers (except stress ulcers), think pain. Imagine a drop of hydrochloric acid on your open hand! First, the hand will hurt or burn, and once the acid has eaten the skin away, the hand will bleed. If the hand could be protected by a glove (food or drugs) the HCL might not eat through enough to bleed.

Drug timing is important in preventing this pain and bleeding. Generally, use anticholinergics before meals. (Refer to **Anticholinergics**.) Tagamet and zantac may be given with or after meals. Consider coating the stomach lining with the "white chalky stuff" such as maalox, titrilac, gelusil, or amphojel 1 hour after meals. Avoid giving within 1 to 2 hours of other medicines. Remind clients on sodium restriction to check the labels for sodium content. Amphojel, titralac, and digel have high sodium content. These clients will also need assistance in dietary modifications.

The Heliocobactor Pylori (Helicopter) organism is prevelent in PUD and can be treated with drugs.

ULCERS

Pain

Ulcers bleed

Drug timing

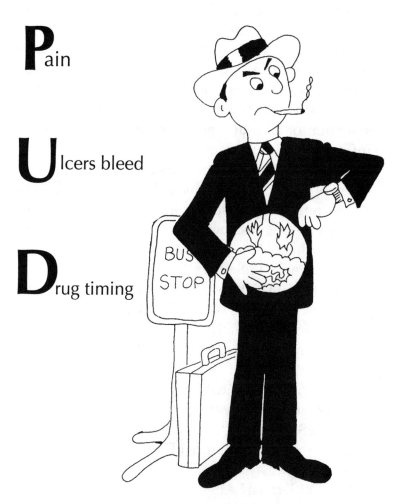

Reprinted with permission ©1994 Nursing Education Consultants

GASTRIC REFLUX

As you can see, *GERD* is holding his stomach due to his problem with gastroesophageal reflux disease (GERD). He is also covering his mouth due to his discomfort with regurgitation of fluid and food particles. GERD is experiencing **REFLUX** of the stomach and duodenal contents into the esophagus leading to a spectrum of clinical manifestations predominated by inflammation of the esophagus.

REFLUX is most often related to inadequate relaxation of the lower esophageal sphincter (LES) that allows reflux of gastric acid and pepsin into the distal esophagus. Agents such as alcohol, benzodiazepines, calcium channel blockers, chocolate, peppermint, and narcotics cause LES relaxation.

REGURGITATION can be decreased by weight reduction if client is obese. The head of the bed may also be elevated. Alterations in the amount of **FOOD** eaten at one serving can also be effective in decreasing reflux. GERD should avoid large meals and sit upright 30–60 minutes after eating. GERD should **X** out carbonated beverages particularly 3 hours prior to going to bed. **ESOPHAGEAL SPASMS** may be relieved by avoiding agents that cause LES relaxation as indicated in the previous paragraph. As you can see, GERD's **LIFESTYLE** must be modified.

Remember GERD must manage this reflux, so he doesn't develop complications with nocturnal aspiration, recurrent pneumonia or bronchospasm, difficulty swallowing, or iron deficiency anemia.

REFLUX

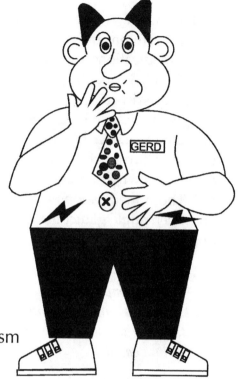

© 2002 I CAN Publishing, Inc.

R egurgitation

E sophageal spasm

F ood—small meals

L ifestyle must be modified

U se of Prilosec, Prevacid, Nexium, Reglan, antacids, H_2 histamine antagonists

X out colas, milk to decrease acid production, peppermint

ANTICHOLINERGICS

The major side effects of these medications are easily seen on the next page. Some examples of these medications include: Atropine, Methantheline (Banthine), Propantheline (Pro-Banthine), and Dicyclomine hydrochloride (Bentyl). Of course these drugs are given because of the desirable effects of decreasing salivation, lacrimation, urination, diarrhea, and GI motility. Blurred vision and dilated pupils are also side effects. It's when we get too much that we get in trouble. These medications are contraindicated in closed and open angle glaucoma, prostatic hypertrophy, and obstructive bowel disease.

Remember – Other current common medications often used for GI symptoms include: Rolaids, Tums, H₂ Antagonists, Proton pump inhibitors, and Helicobacter Pylori agents. Some of the agents are aluminum based and some magnesium based.

ANTICHOLINERGIC MEDICATIONS

Can't pee

Can't see

Can't spit

Can't sh*t

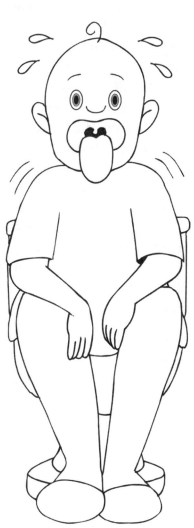

ANTACIDS

Mag has had a history of an ulcer, but feels much better now since antacids coat her stomach lining. She, however, has developed another serious problem with DIARRHEA!!!! This is a major side effect of antacids containing magnesium such as Milk of Magnesia. The diarrhea must get under control or she will need to meet Alkali, a cousin, which will assist her in correcting the metabolic acidosis which may occur as a complication from the diarrhea. **Mag** should be monitored for dehydration, hypokalemia, and hyponatremia. If **Mag** were to remain on magnesium oxide for prolonged therapy, the magnesium level should be monitored periodically.

Al is also in the family and is taking an aluminum antacid such as amphogel for his ulcer symptoms. As you can see, **Al's** problem is constipation. He is so full of it that he can't get rid of it. CONSTIPATION is a major side effect of antacids containing aluminum.

Remember—Teach clients to take antacids one hour after meals and to refrain from taking other oral medications within 1-2 hours of any antacid.

AUNT ACID'S FAMILY

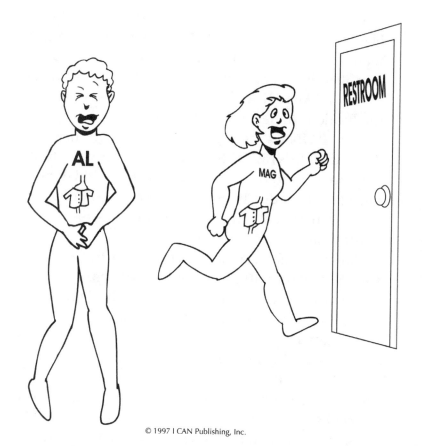

© 1997 I CAN Publishing, Inc.

ALUMINUM   **MA**G**NESIUM**

TREATMENT OF ULCERATIVE COLITIS AND CROHN'S

Cathy Crampy has inflammatory bowel disease. She is bent over with the **CRAMPS** due to the inflammation. This is treated with steroids and a low fat and low fiber diet. Poor Cathy has her legs together to hold in that **DIARRHEA**. She is taking some antidiarrheal medications to decrease this problem.

Her **PAIN** is being relieved through her diet, **ANTICHOLINERGICS** and corticosteroids. Cathy may be NPO to decrease bowel activity; FLUIDS are introduced gradually. She will receive IV fluids and may even require hyperalimentation to restore the deficiencies.

Sulfasalazine (**AZULFIDINE**) is one of the **ANTIMICROBIALS** used to prevent exacerbations.

Her MEALS are modified to correct the deficiencies. She is on a high protein, high caloric and high vitamin diet. Cathy may live a very stressful life. She is always a day behind her deadlines.

COUNSELING will help her to identify how this life style can contribute to this condition. Emotional **SUPPORT** will assist Cathy Crampy in decreasing the stress in her life and help her to learn "To slow down and stop and smell the flowers in life."

CRAMPS

Control diarrhea
Control inflammation

Relieve pain
Restore fluid

Anticholinergics
Antimicrobials

© 1994 I CAN Publishing, Inc.

Meals—correct
nutritional deficiencies

Psychological counseling

Support emotionally/coping

COLOSTOMY

Clients with ulcerative colitis, Crohn's disease or other disease process in the lower gastrointestinal tract may require surgery that brings fecal elimination to an opening on the outside of the abdominal wall.

Connie Colostomy says that her colostomy is just like her **ANUS**.

A   **ABLE** to regulate her stool through regular irrigations; therefore a colostomy bag is not required. Irrigations should be the same time frame daily.

N   **NOT** watery. The stools are formed and do not leak on her clothes.

U   U can do all you can do without the colostomy. Some foods will liquefy stools or cause noisy problems.

S   **SWIMMING** is OK! Showers and tub baths are also acceptable.

This is probably NOT the case for Connie's friend ILLE who has an ileostomy.

Ille's stool is liquid. Bags are attached to the skin and skin breaks down easily. She must be taught about cleaning, removing the adhesive that holds the bag in place and cleanliness of the bag. She is usually not able to regulate the ileostomy because it is watery. She may lose fluids and electrolytes and need replacement. Some foods may also cause noisy (flatus) and "smelly" problems for Ille, which is embarrassing and hard to control.

Remember—Both Connie and Ille will have to live with these ostomys. The nurse's best approach is psychological support and education. They will need support through excellent therapeutic communication. The more they know about caring for themselves, the more "normal" they can be.

CONNIE COLOSTOMY

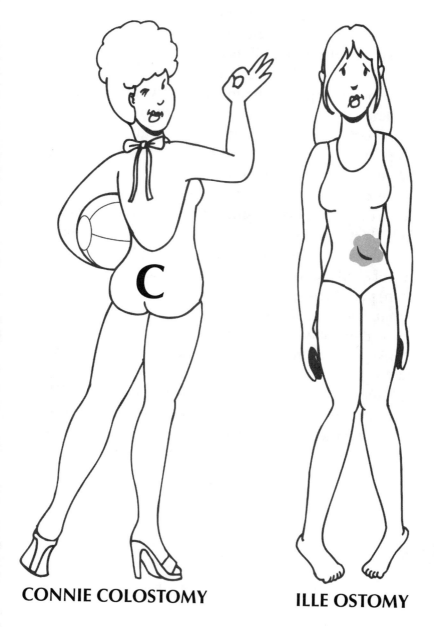

CONNIE COLOSTOMY　　　　**ILLE OSTOMY**

DUMPING SYNDROME

This is a complication that can occur after gastric resection when stomach contents enter the intestine. The image that will pull this concept together for you is the DUMP TRUCK. Imagine that you are in a dump truck on the edge of a mountain. How would you feel? We know we would be nervous as kittens, sweaty and our heart would beat very rapidly. On a mountain edge, we are sure we would be dizzy and very weak. We may also have some abdominal cramping with some distention. These signs are, of course, because we are in the **HIGH** position. (Think of TOO MUCH, TOO SOON = TOO HIGH) Too much carbohydrate, salt, liquid, refined sugar, and in the high position on top of all of that is going to make us (excuse the expression) poop! The gastric contents high in carbohydrates rapidly enter the jejunum.

To remember how to prevent this from occurring, think of the dump truck in the **LOW** position. Think LOW. Teach clients to think small (LOW) meals. The carbohydrates, salt intake, and sugar need to be LOW (small amounts). No fluids with meals or for one hour following the meal. Lie client down for 20 to 30 minutes after meals to delay stomach emptying.

DUMPING SYNDROME

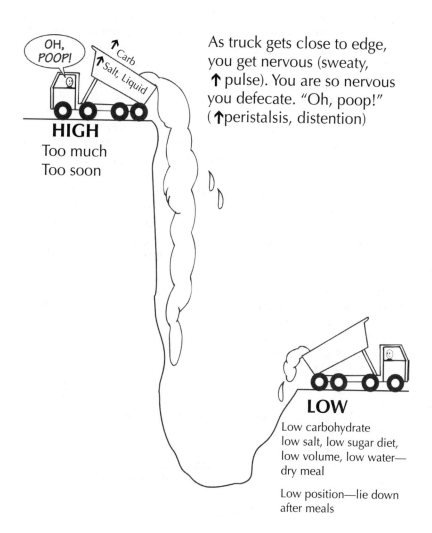

HIGH
Too much
Too soon

As truck gets close to edge, you get nervous (sweaty, ↑ pulse). You are so nervous you defecate. "Oh, poop!" (↑peristalsis, distention)

LOW

Low carbohydrate
low salt, low sugar diet,
low volume, low water—
dry meal

Low position—lie down
after meals

TUBES

First think about the concept of tubes in general. Remember, fluid or air can flow either way in the tube. Usually it is crucial for clients that the material in the tubes flows only the way that it is designed to flow. If it does not, then there can be disastrous results. This disaster most often takes the form of an INFECTION.

Look at a JP (Jackson Pratt) tube for example. This tube is a suction tube designed to suck out or pull off drainage from a specific area. It is imperative that the nurse know the reason for the tubes placement so that she can do some clinical reasoning. We want to be very careful that none of the drainage that it is coming out of the JP tube returns to the wound as this is likely to cause the clinical symptoms of infection in the client.

Let's just take a chest tube for example. The chest has a negative pressure (less than atmospheric). When a sharp knife or other trauma punctures the chest, air is sucked into the chest cavity and causes the lung tissue to collapse. The chest tube is placed into the cavity to renew the negative pressure, but unless the distal end of the tube is under water, the air can still go back into the chest allowing further lung collapse. If we know this, we will do all possible to see that the end of that chest tube stays under water and that we know what emergency measure to take if the water container gets broken.

Another example is the Foley catheter that indwells in the urinary bladder. The urine is "supposed to" flow into a collection bag that is below the level of the bladder. If for any reason that collection bag is moved higher than the level of the bladder, the old collected urine goes back into the bladder and causes an INFECTION.

Clients who are hospitalized and many at home have many tubes inserted into various orifices. It is our responsibility to know the placement and purpose so that we can reason how to care for them.

*Remember **NAVEL** can go into any orifice!*

Narcan
Atropine
Valium
Epinepherine
Lidocaine

TUBES

T rach (nasal, oral) medication

U rinary (foley, supra pubic) medication

B ronchial (chest) medication

E pigastric (nasogastric, JP, feeding, peg) medication

S urgical (drains, CSF drains)

POST-OPERATIVE GI ASSESSMENT

Back in the operating room as a client is being prepared for abdominal surgery, drapes are used over the body to help maintain sterility. Let's use the word **DRAPES** to look at the concept of postoperative GI assessment.

D **DRESSING**–Evaluate amount and characteristics of drainage.

R **RESPIRATORY SYSTEM**–Listen for those breath sounds! Get in some T, C & DB (turning, coughing and deep breathing) to prevent atelectasis.

A *ABDOMINAL ASSESSMENT*–Watch for abdominal distention. Normal bowel sounds should be heard every 5 to 20 seconds. The abdomen should remain soft. If it becomes hard, this may indicate bleeding, paralytic ileus, or peritonitis. If in doubt, measure abdominal girth.

AMBULATE–Will decrease blood clots caused by pooling of blood in extremities. Will decrease the development of a paralytic ileus.

P **PAIN MEDICINE**–Keep them comfortable. If they have a patient-controlled analgesia (PCA) pump in place, teach them how to use it.

PATENCY OF TUBES–This can be done through irrigations and monitoring the suction of drains and tubes.

E **ELIMINATION**– Keep an I & O record.

S **SPLINT**– Splint abdominal incision during T, C, and DB.

GI ASSESSMENT

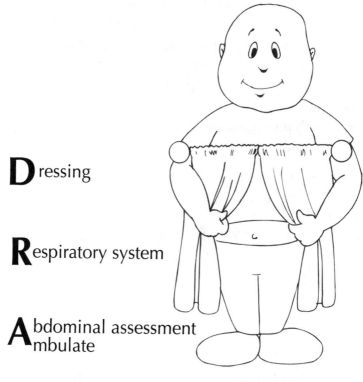

D ressing

R espiratory system

A bdominal assessment
mbulate

© 1994 I CAN Publishing, Inc.

P ain medicine
atency of the tubes

E limination

S plint

ELEVATED LIVER ENZYMES

Remembering elevated liver enzymes is as easy as **ABC**. The next page will assist you with this. When the client has a history of alcoholism, the **ast** and **alt** will be elevated. If the client has a medical problem with biliary obstruction the alp will be elevated. Remember there is a **p** in **alp** and he is *"plugged up Paul."* In clients with a diagnosis of cirrhosis, the ast and alt will be elevated.

A note to remember: These liver enzymes are indicators of liver damage and are utilized as a system specific assessment.

The AST/SGOT normal is 5-40u/L.
The ALT/SGPT normal is 7-56u/L.

ELEVATED LIVER ENZYMES

Remember, elevated liver enzymes are as easy as **ABC**

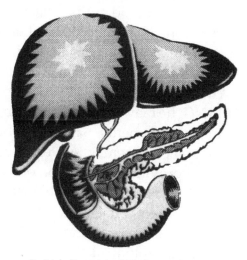

Reprinted with permission ©1994 Creative Educators

A lcoholism (ast, alt)

B iliary obstruction (al**p**) "plugged up Paul"

C irrhosis (ast, alt)

CIRRHOSIS

Here is Larry Leak Liver, who is no longer able to synthesize protein. This results in a decreased colloidal osmotic pressure. (COP holds fluid in the liver and blood vessels.) Since he no longer easily accepts blood from his unique dual blood supply, he also develops portal hypertension. This causes poor Larry to Leak fluid into the peritoneal cavity resulting in **ASCITES**. Too much swelling in the esophagus will cause Larry to get into **AIRWAY** trouble. To prevent complications from **SWELLING**, he may be started on diuretics along with potassium supplements. Salt-poor albumin will assist with hypoalbuminemia. An esophageal tamponade tube will provide compression of **BLEEDING** on esophageal **VARICES**. Prevent bleeding by soft, nonirritating foods. Let's not give him hot coffee to drink. **LABS** such as liver enzymes will be increased. Hypoalbuminemia, prolonged PT, and altered bilirubin metabolism will be seen in lab reports. Hepatic **ENCEPHALOPATHY** will result if Larry is unable to detoxify ammonia, the end product of protein metabolism. As waste products back up, Larry's **SKIN** will turn jaundiced. Decrease discomfort from pruritus. IS THERE HELP? Avoid cocktails (ETOH) and avoid over-the-counter drugs. Larry's liver is simply unable to detoxify them!

CIRRHOSIS

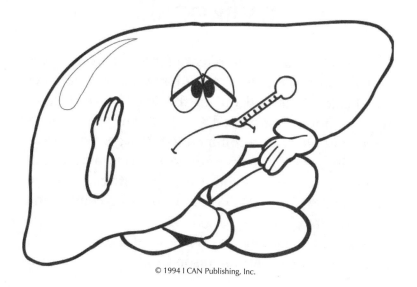

Airway—avoid ETOH and OTC drugs

Swelling

vari**C**es

Inspect lab work

To prevent bleeding

Encephalopathy

Skin

TYLENOL (ACETAMINOPHEN) OVERDOSE

A major undesirable effect of tylenol overdose is hepatic necrosis. It is like we have taken a hammer and beaten "the hell out of the liver." The dose of tylenol should not exceed 4g/day. Other side effects are negligible with recommended dosage. With acute poisoning, the following adverse effects may occur: **anorexia, nausea and vomiting, epigastric** or **abdominal pain, HEPATOTOXICITY, hypoglycemia,** and **hepatic coma**.

Tylenol (Acetaminophen) is a very useful drug for pain and fever. (Refer to Poison Control for more specific plans.)

Remember–Do not administer to clients with liver disease.

TYLENOL OVERDOSE

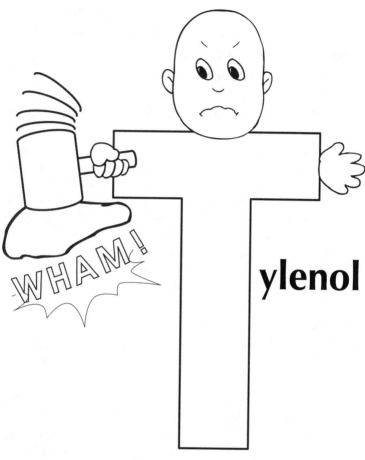

ylenol

PANCREATITIS

The Ace is the high card in a deck of playing cards. This will help you to remember that the "**ASES**" (enzymes of amylase and lipase) are elevated (HIGH) when pancreatitis is present.

P **PAIN MANAGEMENT**–Nonnarcotic analgesics (aspirin, ibuprofen, acetaminophen) may be tried.

PANCREATIC ENZYME replacement therapy may be indicated.

A **ABDOMINAL PAIN**–Typically, acute pancreatitis produces constant epigastric, periumbilical, or left or right upper abdominal pain radiating to the back, often increased by food and decreased by upright posture. Abdominal tenderness, decreased bowel sounds, distention, and fever may be part of the assessment.

N **NPO** initially–Nasogastric suction for exacerbations, Total Parental Nutrition (TPN) and fluid replacement as necessary. Initiate dietary and insulin therapy for diabetes mellitus secondary to pancreatic insufficiency.

C **CALCIUM** may be low.

R **RISK FACTORS**–Alcoholism, biliary tract disease, a penetrating duodenal ulcer and trauma are also associated with pancreatitis.

E **EVALUATE** glucose, electrolytes, hematocrit, serum amylase and lipase, hypotension, and bowel function.

A **ANALGESICS, ANTICHOLINERGICS, ANTACIDS,** *H2-receptor* **ANTAGONISTS, AND ANTIBIOTICS** are utilized.

S **STIMULANTS** such as spices, alcohol, or coffee should be avoided.

PANCREATITIS

"ASES" HIGH

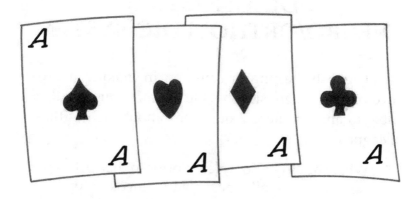

AMYLASE AND LIPASE ARE HIGH WHEN PANCREATITIS IS PRESENT

NEURO /
ORTHOPEDIC SYSTEM

DIAGNOSTICS
NEURO/ORTHOPEDIC SYSTEM

Diagnostic testing is common in making neuro/ orthopedic diagnosis possible. A safe nurse will be able to answer these 3 questions about each of these Diagnostic Tests.

1. What should be completed prior to this test? (consent, teaching, allergies, holding meds or food)?
2. What should happen during this test (positioning, anesthesia, invasive/noninvasive)?
3. What should happen after this test (reporting, monitoring)?

EEG—electroencephalogram used to detect electrical activity of the brain. Noninvasive, wash hair prior to test. Avoid caffeine, energy drink, sedatives.

CT Scan with contrast. Watch for metal. Iodine is often the contrast. Question about stopping metformin (glucophage) before and after test.

Watch for allergies to seafood. Determine contrast to be utilized so that allergies can be assessed.

PET Scan—imaging helps determine organ functioning using radioactive materials. No metal, food or drink containing sugar. Utilizes iodine, assess allergy to seafood.

DIAGNOSTICS
NEURO/ORTHOPEDIC SYSTEM

Remember: Diagnostic exams can be hazardous to the health of our clients.

It is our mission to keep them safe.

The results of these exams are assessments that provide vital information for our critical thinking and clinical reasoning.

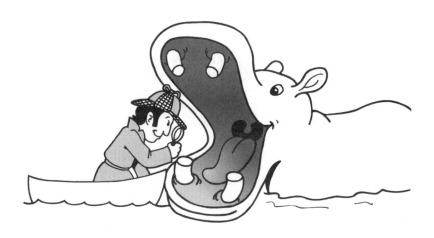

MENINGOCELE/ OMPHALOCELE

Both of these disorders have a sac on the outside of the body. The meningocele is a sac-like cyst of meninges filled with spinal fluid that protrudes through a defect in the bony part of the spine. A myelomeningocele is a sac-like cyst containing meninges, spinal fluid and a portion of the spinal cord with its nerves that protrudes through a defect in the vertebral column. The omphalocele is a protrusion of the intestines on the abdomen.

The nursing care is similar to a seal (**CELE**) in the water. We certainly do not want these sacs (**CELES**) to get too dry. Sterile, normal saline soaks may be used to prevent drying.

Correct positioning is also of paramount importance in preventing damage to the sac (**CELE**) as well as providing nursing care after surgery.

BE KIND TO NATURE AND KEEP THE SEALS IN THE WATER.

MENINGOCELE/OMPHALOCELE

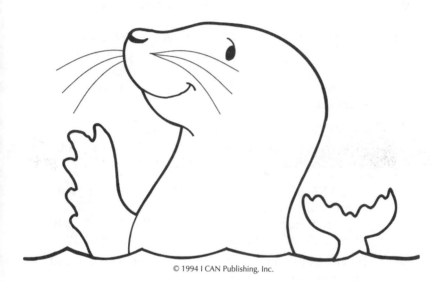

© 1994 I CAN Publishing, Inc.

HYDROCEPHALUS (PIES)

Hydrocephalus is caused by an imbalance in the production and absorption of cerebral spinal fluid (CSF) in the ventricles of the brain. This infant will present with an enlarged head. Visualize **PIES** as we refer to the assessments and plans for this condition.

P   **PROJECTILE VOMITING**–A symptom of increased intracranial pressure (IICP). Teach parents signs of IICP. Many of these infants are difficult to feed, so small feedings at frequent intervals are recommended.

I   **IRRITABILITY**–High pitched cry is characteristic of IICP with an infant. Evaluate the level of consciousness; it is frequently the initial symptom of IICP.

E   **ENLARGED HEAD AND FONTANEL**–Normally at birth, the occipital frontal circumference (OFC) is approximately 2–3 cm. larger than the chest circumference. A bulging fontanel is also a sign of IICP.

     EDUCATE family and refer to appropriate community agencies.

S   **SEPARATION OF SKULL**–As the CSF increases in the ventricles, there will be a separation of the cranial suture lines. They may have bulging "sunset eyes." If infant has a **SHUNT**, observe for infection and IICP.

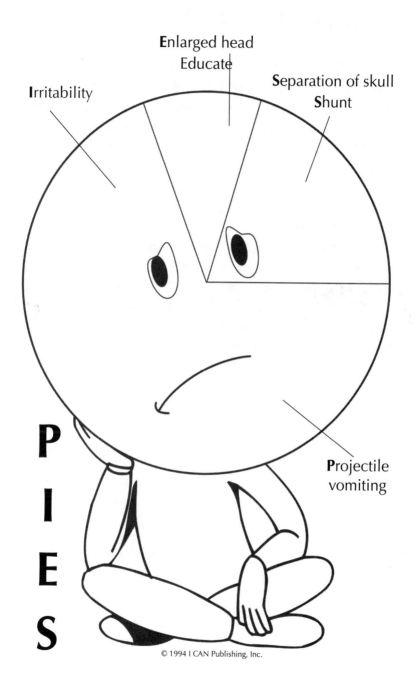

Enlarged head
Educate

Separation of skull
Shunt

Irritability

Projectile
vomiting

P
I
E
S

GLASGOW COMA SCALE

GLASGOW COMA SCALE is often found on both nursing exams and physician orders. In the past this scale has been hard to remember, but here's help. Notice that Glasgow is running (a motor runs, indicating **MOTOR** movements in the client). See Glasgow's **EYES** are open (the client can open eyes on command). The **VERBAL** indicator, like the newspaper comics, lets you know that Glasgow is talking (the client has clear verbal ability).

The score for this scale may range from 3–15. The less responsive, the lower the score; the more responsive, the higher the score.

This is a great scale to evaluate the client's level of consciousness! In summary, the Glasgow Coma Scale evaluates motor, eye opening, and verbal ability.

GLASGOW COMA SCALE

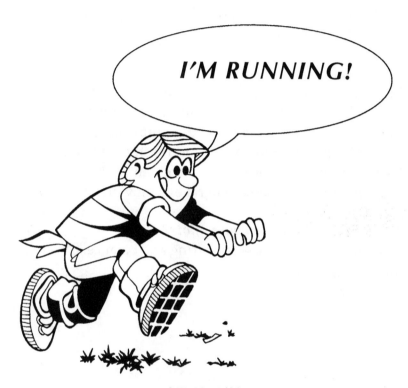

1. MOTOR
2. VERBAL
3. EYES OPEN

CRANIAL NERVES
(3, 4, 6, AND 8)

This tool will help you to remember how some of the cranial nerves may be assessed.

3, 4, 6, makes my eyes do tricks!
Cranial nerves III, IV, and VI (oculomoter, trochlear, and abducens) assess extraocular movements.
Cranial nerve III is assessed by pupil constriction. Assess for pupils being equal and reactive to light.
Cranial nerve IV assesses eye movement.
Cranial nerve VI assesses lateral eye movement.

3, 4, 6, 8, how do we accommodate?
Cranial nerve VIII assesses hearing and balance. Check for hearing acuity.

3, 4, 6, 8

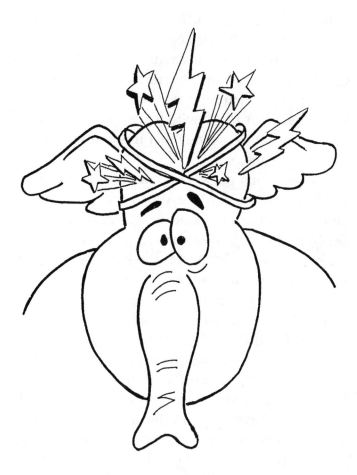

CRANIAL NERVES

Many students find it difficult to remember all 12 of the cranial nerves. This strategy has been developed to simplify the ability to easily remember all 12 of these nerves. Notice that on the next page we only have one nose (*olfactory*), which represents the 1st cranial nerve. God gave us 2 eyes to see with (*optic*), which is the 2nd cranial nerve. I always remember this cranial nerve by recalling "optic vision."

On the previous page, you may recall that cranial nerves 3, 4, 6 makes your eyes do tricks (*oculomotor, trochlear, and abducens*). The 5th cranial nerve is recalled by remembering 5 rhymes with tri (*trigeminal*).

The 7th cranial nerve (*facial*) can be remembered by visualizing placing the number 7 across your face with the top of the 7 going across your forehead and the bottom part going down over your face.

Think of the number 8 (acoustic) fitting nicely into your ear for remembering this nerve. Note that when you evaluate cranial nerves 9 and 10 this assessment is under your chin (*glossopharyngeal and vagus*). Notice these 2 nerves have a "**g**" in the spelling, and one of the assessments for these nerves is to check the **gag** reflex. As you progress to the 11th cranial nerve (*spinal accessory*), visualize a "1" on each shoulder that should remain in place as the client shrugs their shoulder. For the 12th cranial nerve (*hypoglossal*), visualize the client sticking their tongue out from side to side and saying "the end."

CRANIAL NERVES

1 God gave us one nose (olfactory)	**2** God gave us 2 eyes to see with (optic)	**3,4,6** Makes my eyes do tricks! (oculomotor, trochlear, abducens)
5 *TRI* Rhymes with Tri (for Trigeminal)	**7** Can fit nicely across your face to help you remember the Facial Cranial nerves	**8** Fits nicely into your ear to assist you to remember the acoustic
9, 10 Is under my chin. (glossopharyngeal, vagus)	**11** Put a 1 on each shoulder and then shrug them, The 1's should not fall off (spinal accessory)	**12** For tongue movement (hypoglossal)

NEUROLOGICAL CHECKS

There has been a lot of mystery around "neuro checks." The bottom line here is that the client remains alert and oriented, the pupils are equal and reactive to light, and all extremities can move on command. Of course, you want to compare with the last time the neuro checks were done. Were the pupils equal and reactive to light? Were all extremities moving spontaneously and to command? PERL MAE is just lying there in her oyster with one side waving her arm and leg while the other side is limp. Observe that one of her pupils is larger than the other.

These assessments are crucial for any neurological client. Observe the subtle differences! For example, is the client more difficult to arouse than earlier? Your response to this change in assessments can mean the difference between a successful or an unsuccessful recovery!

PERL MAE

Pupils **E**qual **R**eactive to **L**ight
Moving **A**ll **E**xtremities to command

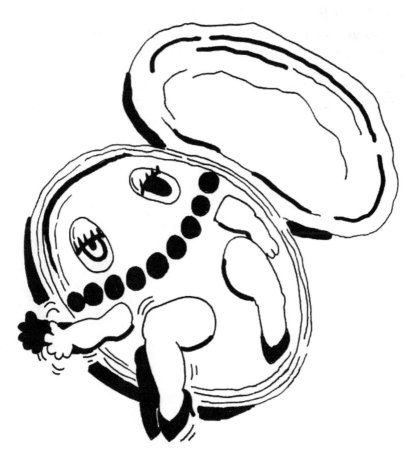

VITAL SIGNS
FOR SHOCK VS. IICP

Most of us have had the vital signs of shock drilled into our heads. We just have a hard time remembering how those vital signs change with increased intracranial pressure (IICP). Guess what? Vital signs in IICP change exactly opposite to changes in shock. All you have to remember are the vital sign changes in shock and you have the connection to recall the vital sign changes for IICP. Both shock and IICP have one commonality–both cause a loss of consciousness.

VITAL SIGNS
FOR SHOCK VS. IICP

Shock	Vs.	IICP
↓	B/P	↑
↑	Pulse	↓
↑	Resp	↓
↓	Temp	↑
↓	Pulse Press	↑
↓	LOC	↓

NURSING CARE FOR INCREASED INTRACRANIAL PRESSURE

Nursing care for the clients with increased intracranial pressure is focused on decreasing the pressure and assessing the level of consciousness. For this reason we use the image of **HEADS** as a memory tool.

H   **HOB**–Maintain semi-Fowler's position to promote venous drainage and respiratory function. This would be contraindicated if the client had a spinal cord injury.

E   **EVALUATE NEUROLOGICAL CHECKS**–The first sign of a change in the level of intracranial pressure is an alteration in the level of consciousness. Pupils also should react equally to light.

A   **AIRWAY**–Evaluate current respiratory pattern. May require intubation and control on a volume ventilator.

D   **DRAINAGE**–Drainage from the ears may be cerebral spinal fluid. A CSF leak would test positive for glucose. Apply a sterile dressing over ear and evaluate for signs of meningitis.

S   **SAFETY**–Seizure precautions. No sedatives or narcotics. Restrict fluids. Control temperature, and avoid coughing.

NURSING CARE FOR INCREASED CRANIAL PRESSURE

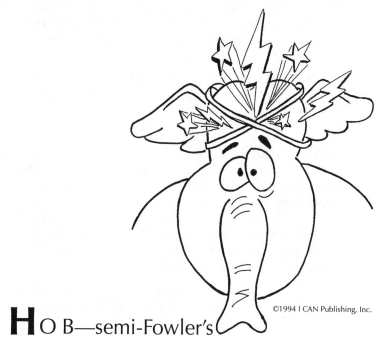

©1994 I CAN Publishing, Inc.

HO B—semi-Fowler's

Evaluate ICP

Airway—oxygen supplement

Drainage

Safety

SEIZURES

Caesar is experiencing an interruption of normal brain functioning by uncontrolled paroxysmal discharge of electrical stimuli from the neurons. **"CAESAR"** will outline the general nursing care for clients with seizures.

C COUNSELING is important for the family and the client to assist them in maintaining positive coping mechanisms.

CALM–After a seizure occurs, maintain a calm atmosphere and provide privacy.

A ANTICONVULSANTS–Phenobarbital (Sodium luminal), Primidone (Mysoline), Carbamazepine (Tegretol), or Phenytoin (Dilantin) are some examples of anticonvulsants.

APNEA and/or cyanosis must be monitored. Do not force anything into the client's mouth if the jaws are clenched shut. If the jaws are not clenched, place an airway in the client's mouth after the seizure. Artificial ventilation cannot be performed on a client during a tonic-clonic seizure.

E EVALUATE changes in the level of consciousness. After the seizure, evaluate client's orientation, activity, and any level of paralysis or muscle weakness.

S SAFETY–Protect the client from injuring himself by falling out of bed or striking himself on bedrails, etc. Loosen any constrictive clothing. Do not restrain client during seizure activity.

A AVOID ALCOHOL.

ACTIVITIES–Identify any activities that occurred immediately prior to the seizure. Describe any activity (movement) that occurred and body area affected.

R REDUCE STIMULI.

REMAIN with the client who is in seizure activity. Note the time the seizure began and how long it lasted.

REORIENT client after the seizure.

Remember–SAFETY is the biggest issue.

CAESAR (SEIZURES)

C
A
E
S
A
R

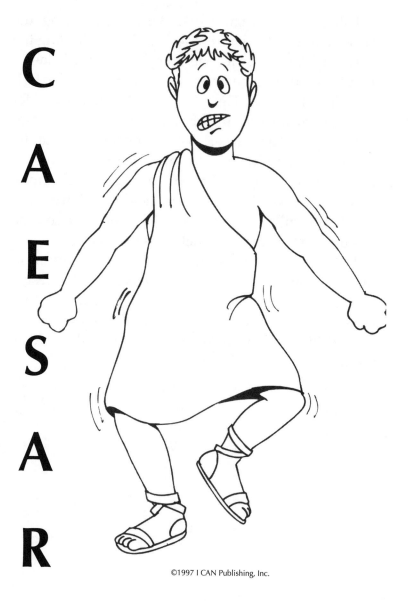

DILANTIN (DIAL AT TEN)

Dilane has a seizure disorder and is taking the drug dilantin. She does not feel well and is calling the nurse at 10:00 a.m. Her therapeutic level for Dilantin should be 10-20 micrograms/ml. (EASY TO REMEMBER. THERE IS A TIN [TEN] IN DILANTIN.) Her adverse reactions from this medication include **gingival hyperplasia**, (see, she's showing you her big gums) **GI disturbances, hepatotoxicity**, (her liver is visible on her abdomen) **ataxia** (her legs are shaking), **hypocalcemia** and a decrease in the absorption of **vitamin D** (the milk on the table and the sunshine coming through the window will help this problem).

If Dilane's level becomes toxic be sure and inform the physician. The medication will likely be decreased. If administered IV, then the only IV fluid that it should be mixed with is normal saline. During infusion, it is a good idea to always keep your eye on the cardiac monitor.

Remember–Teach good oral hygiene and nutrition.

DILANTIN (DIAL AT TEN)

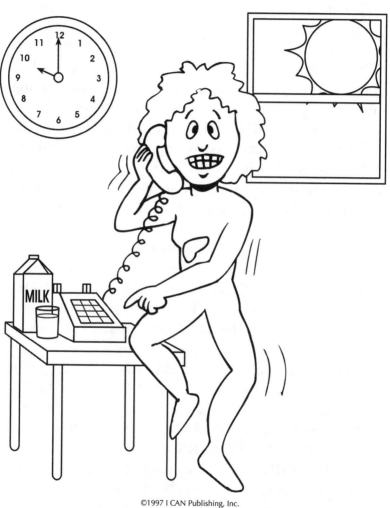

PARKINSON'S DISEASE

Meet **PARK DARK**, our little old man with Parkinson's disease. This condition results from a depletion of, or an imbalance in dopamine and increased activity in acetylcholine.

Park's fingers want to "**PILL ROLL**" all the time. This tremor is rhythmic and rapid. Worse still, when he gets up out of the chair, his bottom is always trying to catch up with his head and never quite makes it, so he is often **ABOUT TO FALL. RIGIDITY** of the muscles results in jerky, uncoordinated "cogwheel" movements. Park is not always the fellow who wants to go to the restaurant for dinner because he "**KAN'T**" **SWALLOW WELL**, DROOLS his food and might get choked.

Park's last name is **Dark** because this is a dark, depressing disease, and he gets very sad about the whole thing. Medications used to enhance **DOPAMINE** secretion are levodopa (L-DOPA) and SINEMET. One of the latest drugs used for Parkinson's Disease is ropinirole (Requip), a non-ergot alkaloid dopamine agonist. **ARTANE** and cogentin are used to decrease effects of acetylcholine. Sometimes **COFFEE RESTRICTION** can reduce the pill rolling. Some ANTIHISTAMINES may be helpful to **KEEP MUSCLE TREMORS DOWN**.

PARK DARK bears watching. He unfortunately falls, spills hot food on himself and can get depressed to the point of harming himself. *He will need your support!*

PARK DARK

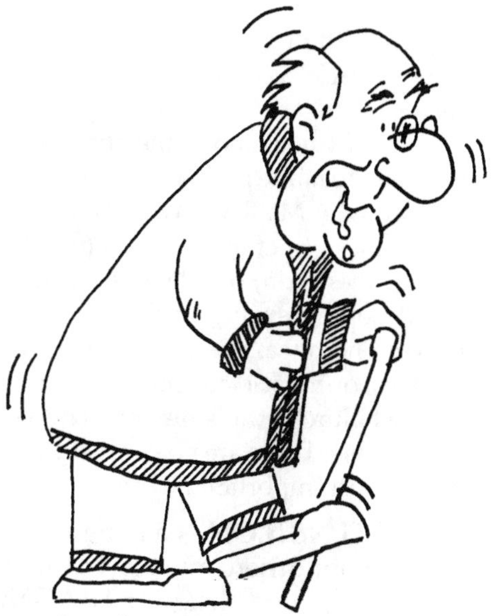

Pill rolling

About to fall

Rigidity

Kan't swallow/speak (drools)

©1994 I CAN Publishing, Inc.

Dopamine/L-Dopa/Sinemet

Artane—improves rigidity

Restrict coffee

Keep tremors down with antihistimine

MYASTHENIA GRAVIS

Why didn't somebody tell us that myasthenia gravis means grave muscle weakness? If they had, we would have asked ourselves where are the muscles? The heart is a muscle.

Muscles help move the chest for breathing and the legs for walking, to name just a few. If there is grave muscle weakness, we can see why **MYRA DYSTONIA** will get into deep trouble fast if she doesn't get her muscle strengthening medication (prostigmin or mestinon) on TIME! As you can see **MYRA DYSTONIA** has drooping eyelids and may even experience some difficulty moving her face. She will NOT have any sensory deficit, loss of reflexes, or muscle atrophy. This progressive weakness is caused from a failure in transmission of nerve impulses due to acetylcholine release. There are no cures at the present time. "**TIME**" is one of the most important factors.

T   **TENSILON** is a drug with a short half life that will strengthen muscle weakness in Myra. This makes it a good drug for DIAGNOSIS and differentiating types of crisis (cholinergic crisis versus myasthenic crisis). It is not routinely given for treatment due to its short term effect.

I   **INFECTION** and exercise make MYRA worse.

M   **MUST** give medications on time. We sure don't want MYRA to go on that ventilator. We MUST avoid the use of sedatives and tranquilizers which cause respiratory depression. We MUST not give the client anything to eat or drink during a myasthenic crisis due to the risk of aspiration. After the crisis, remember to assess the ability to swallow and give a diet which is soft and easily swallowed.

E   **EXACERBATIONS** and remission are part of this experience, but since the weakness is progressive it's likely to get worse with TIME.

MYRA DYSTONIA

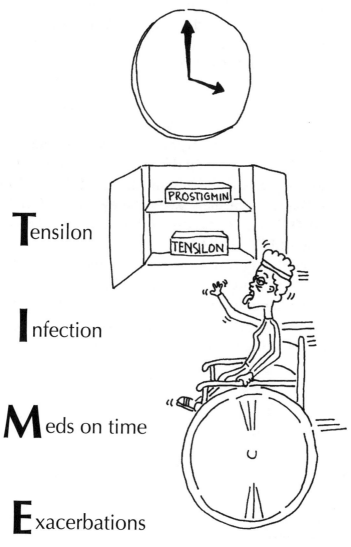

Tensilon

Infection

Meds on time

Exacerbations

BELL'S PALSY

Ring the Bell for the Palsy that affects the seventh cranial nerve, resulting in muscle flaccidity on one side of the face. If the facial appearance is permanent, clients may need counseling assistance with maintaining a positive **IMAGE**. They may be ringing your call bell because of "pain" behind the ear, drooping of the mouth and an eyelid that won't close. **ANALGESICS** will be given to decrease the pain behind the ear. Ophthalmic ointment and eye patches may be needed at night to prevent drying of the cornea on the affected side. During the day, instilling **METHYLCELLULOSE** drops will help keep the eye moist (**GIVE EYE CARE**). Due to the discomfort, **EVALUATE** the client's **ABILITY TO EAT**.

Treatment may consist of corticosteroids and vasodilators. An inability to close the eyelid on the affected side, and a sagging mouth is scary; however, proper treatment and good nursing care will usually help clear up the problem with little residual.

BELL'S PALSY

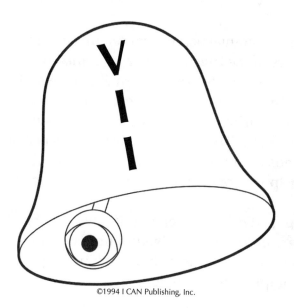

©1994 I CAN Publishing, Inc.

Image

Methylcellulose

Analgesics

Give eye care

Evaluate ability to eat

TRIGEMINAL NEURALGIA (TIC DOULOUREUX)

This is a cranial nerve disorder affecting the sensory branches of the trigeminal nerve (cranial nerve V). Let us introduce you to Luke W. Arm. Luke says, "Hot food is painful!" He has a closed eye from frequent blinking and tearing. Facial twitching and grimacing are characteristic. The pain he experiences is usually brief and ends as abruptly as it begins. The word **"PAINE"** will help you remember the nursing care for Luke W. Arm.

The medical management of pain may be Dilantin or Tegretol, Dilantin, or Neurontin. The surgical intervention is a local nerve block or interruption of the nerve impulse transmission.

TRIGEMINAL NEURALGIA

Pain is excruciating

Avoid hot or cold

Increase protein and calories

Nerve, cranial V

Eye care

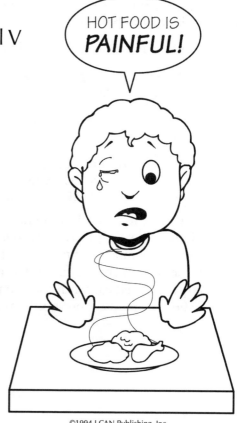

BOTOX

Botulinum is a dangerous organism that can give us food poisoning and can kill us. However, it has been found to be effective in the treatment of many medical disorders if given in very small doses.

The primary purpose of BOTOX is to relax muscles. This very positive action can work wonders in many areas. Because BOTOX allows muscles to relax usually within 3 days, it has become a very important product for cosmetic use in that frown lines and wrinkles disappear.

To be considered a safe practitioner of nursing, we must be aware of the dangers of administering the drug and of the side effects.

B   **Botulinum** is a very poisonous substance and should be monitored carefully.

O   **Occasional** headaches and nausea are side effects.

T   **Target** muscles relax, deleting frown lines, wrinkles and some symptoms of dystonia.

O   **Opening** of the eye may be affected and ptosis may occur.

X   **X** out clients that already have muscle weakness (i.e., myasthenia gravis, cerebral palsy, etc.) as the Botox may affect or weaken non-targeted muscle groups.

Watch out for muscle weakness, especially that affects breathing and seeing! "The **Ox** Relaxing in the **Boat**" will help you remember that to promote client safety the nurse must monitor client for too much relaxation. If the client already has a medical condition that results in muscle weakness, then the medication should not be administered!

BOTOX

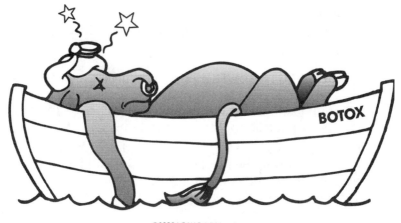

©2008 I CAN Publishing, Inc.

B otulinum

O ccasional headaches and nausea

T arget muscles relax

O pening of the eye may be affected

X out clients who have muscle weakness

ADVERSE EFFECTS OF IMMOBILITY

It is **AWFUL** being immobilized! Have you ever tried it? The nursing goals are to prevent these potential complications from occurring.

A **ATELECTASIS**–There may be a decrease in client's ability to cough and move those secretions which will result in a decreased oxygen exchange. Infections can lead to this complication.

Encourage turning, coughing and deep breathing. Putting the head of the bed up will help with breathing and coughing. Maintain adequate hydration.

W **WASTING OF THE BONES**–Demineralization of bones leads to muscle weakness and atrophy. Range of motion exercises are mandatory. Maintain appropriate alignment while positioning.

F **FUNCTION LOSS**–This can result from the above problem. Prevent by active contracting and relaxing large muscles.

U **URINARY STASIS**–Increase those fluids and decrease the calcium intake. If possible, have client sit to void.

L **LAST BUT NOT LEAST CONSTIPATION**– Encourage diet with adequate protein, bulk and liquids.

IMMOBILITY

Atelectasis

Wasting of bones

Functional loss of muscle

Urinary stasis

Last but not least, constipation

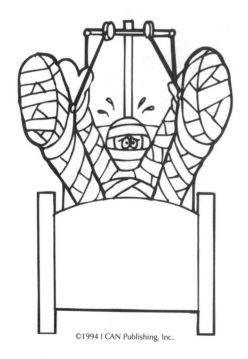

PERIPHERAL VASCULAR DISEASE

V   VENOUS VALVES DEFECTIVE
VEIN WALLS LEAK
VARICOSE VEINS

E   ELEVATE LEGS
W E IGHT REDUCTION

BRAW N Y IN COLOR

T O   PICAL STEROIDS

H OSE

U   ULCERS

S   STANDING A LOT!
SKIN COLOR CHANGES

PERIPHERAL VASCULAR DISEASE

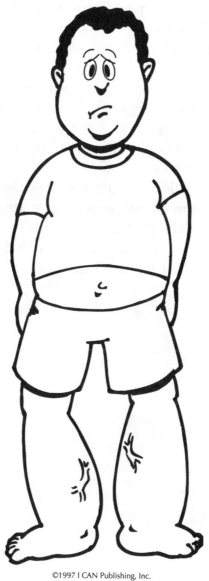

POLYCYTHEMIA

Polycythemia Vera (Primary) is a blood disorder characterized by a proliferation of all red marrow cells. This disorder usually develops in middle ages. Several of the clinical manifestations and diagnostics are outlined below. To assist you in remembering this, just visualize "Mr. Ruddy" on the next page. His complexion looks as if someone had taken a red crayon and colored his face to give him a **ruddy complexion**. He may also present with an **enlarged liver**. Several diagnostics that are prevalent with polycythemia include: an **erythrocyte** count that is **elevated, excessive production of leukocytes and platelets**. Another clinical manifestation that may occur is a **decrease in the blood flow**. Treatment of care includes a phlebotomy and a **decrease in the iron intake**.

POLYCYTHEMIA

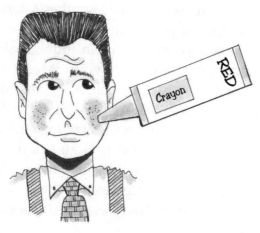

Ruddy complexion

Erythrocytes increased
Excessive production of leukocytes and platelets
Enlarged liver

Decreased blood flow
Decreased iron intake

ALLOPURINOL (ZYLOPRIM)

Allopurinol (Zyloprim) the drug of choice to prevent GOUT decreases uric acid synthesis. Uric acid is the end product of purine metabolism. Condition of hyperuricemia may also occur in individuals receiving chemotherapy (secondary gout). Medications for an acute attack may include colchicine, indomethacin (Indocin) or naproxen (Naprosyn).

Gout is generally rapid with swelling and a painful joint. Typically the uric acid crystals are in the large toe, but may also involve ankles and knees. During an acute attack, protect the affected joint by immobilizing the joint. Encourage gradual weight reduction. Instruct the client to avoid salicylates. Encourage **high fluid intake** (>3L / day) to increase excretion of uric acid and to prevent the development of uric acid stones.

Teach clients to avoid foods high in purines such as **organ meats**, shell fish, and preserved fish (anchovies, sardines) and avoid **alcohol**. We would like to see the urine output **increased** to 2 liters per day to help decrease the risk of stones. Clients at risk for stones may be given trisodium citrate for urine alkalinization.

Remember–Clients with renal insufficiency
should receive a reduced dose of Allopurinol.

ALLOPURINOL (GOUT)

Gulp 3 liters fluid per day

Ø organ meats or wines

Urine output increased to 2 liters per day

Teach

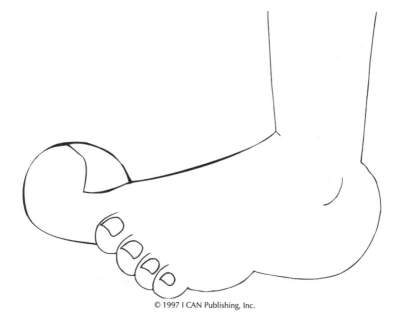

OSTEOPOROSIS

JOSEPHINE BONE-A-PART is working to prevent immobility in her "mature years." She is on a treadmill because weight-bearing exercise increases bone strength. She may also take Fosomax and calcium to decrease her risk of developing osteoporosis. ACTONEL is another prescription that may be used to prevent and treat osteoporosis in post-menopausal women. She knows that her drinking and smoking have got to stop if she doesn't want to be laid up with broken **BONES.**

B BONE density studies are the noninvasive x-ray diagnostic tests that are commonly used. There is no prep, no pain and not much time involved in this x-ray. Just lie down and they'll shoot it.

O OUT of calcium is an issue. Inadequate calcium intake early in life may have predisposed Josephine Bone-A-Part to the development of osteoporosis. Calcium supplemental therapy (about 1500mg per day) is usually recommended for post-menopausal women. Young women should be advised to have a daily dietary intake of at least 1000 to 1500 mg of calcium per day. Magnesium and Vitamin D may also need to be supplemented.

N NEED Drugs **AFTER** osteoporosis has developed and to prevent further deterioration. The drugs on Josephine's table work in different ways. To decrease the GI side effects of most of these medications, drink with 8 ounces of water first thing in the morning. Stay sitting up and NPO for at least half an hour before eating or taking other drugs. Forteo, an expensive injectable drug, is currently used in the treatment of severe osteoporosis.

E ESTROGEN given orally has demonstrated its ability to decrease the incidence of osteoporosis. In addition, estrogen improves the client's lipid profile (HDL cholesterol rises, LDL cholesterol falls) and overall cardiovascular risk declines. Weight bearing EXERCISE, such as walking, helps the BONES. EDUCATION early in life will assist in preventing complications from osteoporosis.

S STRESS fractures especially of the hip, waist or vertebra are common. Education and prevention of falls are important in minimizng fractures and maintaining independence for post-menopausal women.

Remember–Prevention is the BEST action!

JOSEPHINE BONE-A-PART

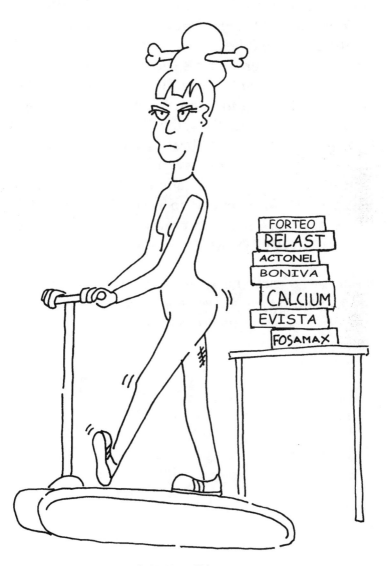

ARTHRITIS

Arthur has osteoarthritis. He wakes up in the morning stiff and achy and finds it hard to reach his walking cane. His fingers are all swollen at the joints (Herberden's nodules) and other joints are affected. He may feel better after his shower as the hot water warms up those joints. Arthur has on his swim trunks because he is going to water therapy at the local spa. Water therapy is probably the best exercise since it better protects his weight bearing joints. He will definitely need to rest after his swim.

Tylenol may be the medication of choice and Arthur will have to be reminded to keep his dosage at or below 4 gms/24 hours to prevent an overdose. (See **TYLENOL OVERDOSE**)

Remember—Arthur may not want to move because of his pain, but physical activity is imperative for him to retain his independence.

ARTHUR ITIS

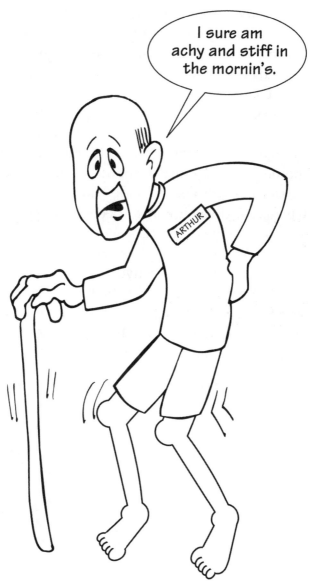

MULTIPLE MYELOMA

Meet "Mr. Bone" who will assist you in remembering the priority information for multiple myeloma. This disorder is a malignancy of the plasma cells, most common in men in their 60's. These malignant cells infiltrate into bones and soft tissues resulting in severe pain to the client.

Clients experience back and bone pain along with anemia and broken bones. Many clients will be on pain medication and comfort measures. Treatment consists of chemotherapy and palliative radiation therapy. Glucocorticosteroids are also included in the treatment plan. Clients need calcitonin to decrease hypercalcemia and reduce bone destruction.

To assist in maintaining physical equilibrium, clients must be encouraged to hydrate, ambulate, and medicate! Clients need to be evaluated for adequate hydration to prevent calcium from precipitating in the kidneys. Careful ambulation is helpful in decreasing hypercalcemia and improving pulmonary status.

Safety measures are necessary to prevent pathologic fractures!

MULTIPLE MYELOMA

Broken bones

On pain medication and chemotherapy

Need calcitonin

Evaluate blood and kidneys
    (will show calcium loss)

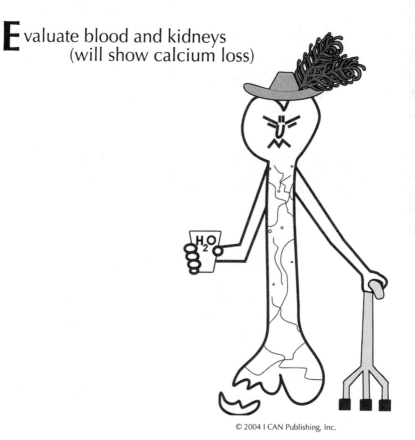

AMBULATE, MEDICATE, HYDRATE

NONSTEROIDAL ANTI-INFLAMMATORY DRUGS (NSAIDS)

NSAIDs are a group of medications that prevent prostaglandin synthesis. What does that mean? Prostaglandins contribute to the following: inflammation, body temperature, pain transmission, platelett aggregation, and other actions. These prostaglandins are not stored, but are released on demand.

What type of physical problems may benefit from NSAIDs? Fever and inflammation (ie. arthritis) can be reduced by these medications.

Are there any undesirable effects from NSAIDs? There are several undesirable effects that the nurse must assess and educate clients to report. These include GI upset or bleeding, **ototoxicity** (ringing in the ears), **hepatic necrosis**, or **nephritis**.

As a nurse, what should be included in the plan of care?

1. Administer medications with **food to decrease GI irritation**.

2. Teach clients about actions and side effects and report any dark, tarry stools, "coffee ground or bloody emesis", other **GI distress or ringing in the ears**.

3. Instruct client to inform health care providers about these medications prior to any dental or other type of surgery. NSAIDs should be discontinued approximately 5–7 days before the procedure to prevent any complications with bleeding.

4. NSAIDs are not the drugs of choice if the client has any compromise in either the renal system or the liver.

5. Evaluate the effectiveness of the NSAIDs.

NSAIDS

No alcohol

Side effects

Aspirin sensitivity—
do not give

Ibuprofen, Indocin, Vioxx
are a few examples

Do take with food

Stop 5–7 days
before surgery

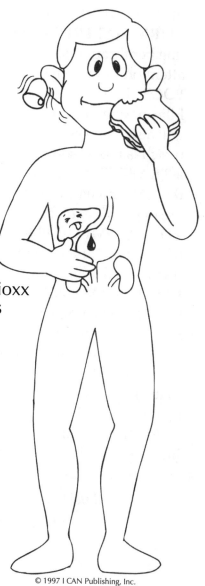

CARE OF CLIENT IN TRACTION

Ellie Elephant gets in more trouble. She has fallen, **FRACTURED** her trunk, and is in traction. We will need a **FIRM MATTRESS**, and will probably need help putting her through **RANGE OF MOTION** exercises. Pay attention to those feet; we don't want a problem with **FOOT DROP**. Without good body **ALIGNMENT**, Ellie may get contractures and decubiti. **ALIGNMENT** will also help keep the traction pulling from both ends which is the reason for traction anyway. Let's get Ellie a **TRAPEZE**, so that she can help us turn her to keep the pneumonia away. Ellie needs to cough and deep breathe on regular intervals to prevent **RESPIRATORY COMPLICATIONS**. One **COMPLICATION** of a fracture of long bones is a fat embolism. It can be transported to the lungs producing symptoms of acute **RESPIRATORY** distress. Now what will we do about her **URINARY** retention? Increase fluid intake. Ellie may need help with the bedpan. Be sure and *evaluate for circulatory impairments*. The 5 P's will help. They are pain, pallor of skin, pulses (especially distal to the injury), paresthesia, and paralysis. Compartmental syndrome can be a major problem.

Another example of traction is a Halo. Priority nursing care includes assessing hardware for stability and signs of infection.

Good Luck! Elephants and people in traction
can be a major challenge!

CARE OF CLIENT IN TRACTION

Firm mattress
oot drop

ROM—for unaffected
extremities

Alignment

Complications

Trapeze

Urinary retention

Respiratory complications

Evaluate circulatory impairments
(5 P's)

CRUTCH WALKING

Remembering how to instruct the client to use crutches while walking up and down the stairs is "INSANELY EASY". Just look at our friend, Charlie, with his crutches on the next page. He is putting his good leg up on the stair first "UP TO HEAVEN!" When he goes down, his bad leg will go first! Remember, "BAD GOES TO YOU KNOW WHERE."

CANE WALKING

These same principles work for the client walking with the cane. The difference is that the cane is used in the opposite hand of the affected limb.

Remember – Strong side leads!

CRUTCH WALKING

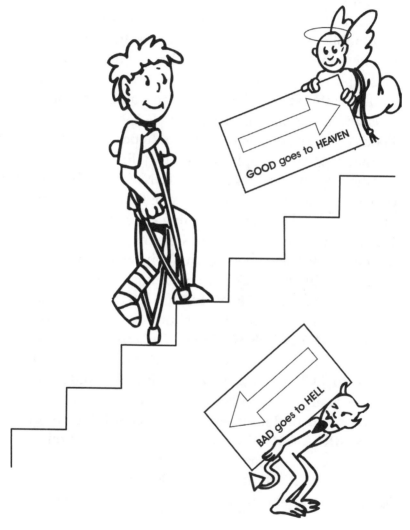

CARE OF THE SPINAL CORD CLIENT

"PARALYZED POOCH" has been out partying with the neighborhood dogs and has been in an automobile accident. He broke his neck and is unfortunately paralyzed from the neck down. The paramedic dog who came to the scene had to access his airway by a "jaw thrust" and log roll him to stabilize his neck. This will minimize further **CORD DAMAGE**. Assess Pooch's breath sounds for signs of hypoxia. Incentive spirometry and chest physiotherapy will assist in optimizing **RESPIRATORY FUNCTION**. Due to his loss of bladder function, **URINARY** retention is a problem. He will either have an indwelling catheter or require intermittent catheterization. Prevent urinary tract infections! Because Pooch is immobile watch for blood clots (**THROMBUS**). Compression stockings may help venous return. **CARDIOVASCULAR STABILITY** can be a problem due to SHOCK or autonomic dysreflexia. (Refer to **AUTONOMIC DYSREFLEXIA**, page 348.)

Pooch needs a **NEURO ASSESSMENT** for IICP (Refer to IICP visual). **FLUIDS AND ROUGHAGE** are necessary to keep bladder and bowels working. Calories and protein need to be increased. Watch for **SKIN BREAKDOWN**. An ounce of prevention is worth a pound of cure. Pooch is going to have a major life change. He will need **SUPPORT** in ventilating his feelings and establishing realistic short-term goals.

Remember, check for the tightness of those screws in the traction.

CARE OF SPINAL CORD CLIENT

Paralysis

A ssess urinary/bowel

R espiratory depression/airway

A ssess neuro/LOC

L og roll

Y our circulation

Z ap out thrombus

E ncourage protein/fluid

D erma tone/dermatology

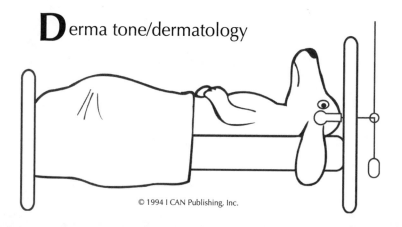

ANTICOAGULANTS

Coumadin, Heparin and Lovenox are used to inhibit thrombus and clot formation. Clotting times will be prolonged which will assist in maintaining the flow or "stream of blood."

The key to successfully remembering the lab reports and antidotes for the appropriate anticoagulants are to think of (H) looking like 2 tt's in Heparin. The lab report necessary to evaluate while clients are on heparin is Ptt. The antidote also has 2 t's in it (protamine sulfate).

Coumadin's antidote is vitamin K. **C** and **K** sound alike which will help with association. The lab report which needs to be monitored is Pt.

Labs now report INR (international normalized ratio) values. The range for most clients on anticoagulants is 2–3. The exceptions are mechanical heart valves and recurrent thromboembolism clients who should be anticoagulated to an INR of 3–4.5.

ANTICOAGULANTS

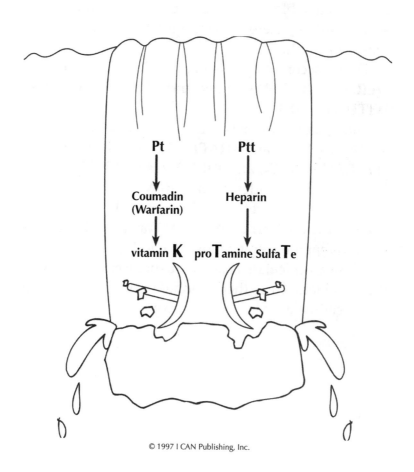

Pt

Ptt

**Coumadin
(Warfarin)**

Heparin

vitamin K

proTamine SulfaTe

AUTONOMIC DYSREFLEXIA

This condition may occur in clients with a spinal cord injury at T_6 or higher. The stimuli below the level of injury triggers the sympathetic nervous system to dump catecholamines resulting in hypertension. Spinal injury blocks the normal transmission of sensory impulses. There is an exaggerated response to the sensory stimuli.

The most common causes are the 3 F's: **FULL BLADDER, FECAL IMPACTION**, and a **FUNNY FEELING WITH THE SKIN**.

The assessments that occur as a result of these causes are: **FLUSHING** and **DIAPHORESIS, HEADACHE, HYPERTENSION**, and **BRADYCARDIA**. The priority treatment is to identify and REMOVE the CAUSE. Frequently the dysreflexia will subside. If possible, the head of the bed can be elevated. Watch the hypertension, so that it doesn't get out of hand.

These folks feel real bad and usually cannot tell you their problem. Once their bladder or bowel is emptied the sweating and bad feelings go away.

AUTONOMIC DYSREFLEXIA (INJURIES AT T_6 OR HIGHER

Causes
1. Full bladder
2. Fecal impaction
3. Funny feeling with the skin

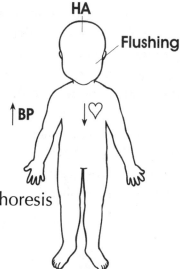

Assessments
1. Flushing & Diaphoresis
2. Headache
3. Hypertension
4. Bradycardia

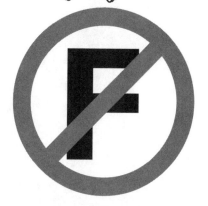

STROKE

When blood flow to the brain is interrupted, the assessment is an emergency. The American Heart Association utilizes the acronym "FAST" to help with the original assessment. If any of the assessments are deficient, the client must immediately reach medical help. Treatment that begins within 3 hours of the incident has the best chance for brain survival.

The treatment depends on the medical diagnosis of an ischemic incident or a brain bleed. If no hemorrhage is found, clot busting drugs such as tPA (tissue plasminogen activation) are usually administered. "FAST" becomes even more important when nurses realize the tPA is often ineffective if administered longer than 3 hours after the original incident.

Migraine headaches can mimic the symptoms of a stroke (CVA). Assessments are of paramount importance with these system specific assessments to prevent long range complications.

CVA

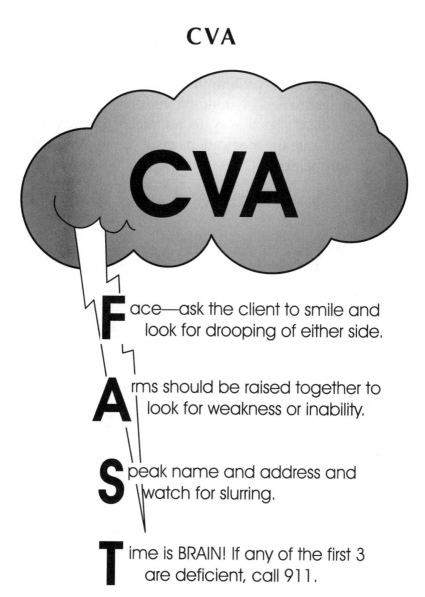

F ace—ask the client to smile and look for drooping of either side.

A rms should be raised together to look for weakness or inability.

S peak name and address and watch for slurring.

T ime is BRAIN! If any of the first 3 are deficient, call 911.

®2011 I CAN Publishing®, Inc.

*Remember, we only have 3 hours! Be **FAST** in assessments.*

MAGIC 2'S

The magician is pulling the prescription drugs out of his magic hat and reminding you that you can use the"MAGIC 2's"as a way to remember the toxicity level. These are the medications most commonly monitored for therapeutic dosage.

MONITORING DRUGS BY THE MAGIC 2'S

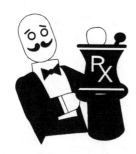

Drug	Range	Toxicity
Digitalis	.5-1.5	**2**
Lithium	.6-1.2	**2**
Aminophylline (Theophylline)	10-20	**20**
Dilantin	10-20	**20**
Acetaminophen	1-30	**200**

THE MAGIC 4'S

Sometimes it's hard to remember those electrolyte extracellular levels; however, we MUST because they affect the heart as recorded by the EKG. The digit **4** can be magic in helping to remember. Even though not electrolytes, the hemoglobin and hematocrit can also be remembered using a **4**. For example if the hemoglobin is **14** the hematocrit will be **42**. The pH, pCO_2, and HCO_3, may also be difficult to remember until you review the **MAGIC 4's**.

THE MAGIC 4'S

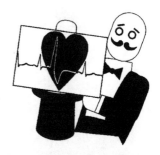

Electrolyte	Range	Magic 4
K	3.5–5.5	**4**
Cl	98–106	10**4**
Na	135–145	1**4**0
pH	7.34–7.45	7.**4**0
pCO$_2$	35–45	**4**0
HCO$_3$	22–26	2**4**

INDEX

Note: Page numbers in italics refer to images.

NOTES

NOTES

NOTES

NOTES

NOTES

NOTES